Reflective Practice in Nursing

Transforming Nursing Practice series

Transforming Nursing Practice is the first series of books designed to help students meet the requirements of the NMC Standards and Essential Skills Clusters for degree programmes. Each book addresses a core topic, and together they cover the generic knowledge required for all fields of practice. Accessible and challenging, *Transforming Nursing Practice* helps nursing students prepare for the demands of future healthcare delivery.

Core knowledge titles:

Series editor: Professor Shirley Bach, Head of the School of Nursing and Midwifery at the University of Brighton

Acute and Critical Care in Adult Nursing	ISBN 978 0 85725 842 7
Becoming a Registered Nurse: Making the Transition to Practice	ISBN 978 0 85725 931 8
Communication and Interpersonal Skills in Nursing (2nd edn)	ISBN 978 0 85725 449 8
Contexts of Contemporary Nursing (2nd edn)	ISBN 978 1 84445 374 0
Dementia Care in Nursing	ISBN 978 0 85725 873 1
Getting into Nursing	ISBN 978 0 85725 895 3
Health Promotion and Public Health for Nursing Students	ISBN 978 0 85725 437 5
Introduction to Medicines Management in Nursing	ISBN 978 1 84445 845 5
Law and Professional Issues in Nursing (2nd edn)	ISBN 978 1 84445 372 6
Leadership, Management and Team Working in Nursing	ISBN 978 0 85725 453 5
Learning Skills for Nursing Students	ISBN 978 1 84445 376 4
Medicines Management in Adult Nursing	ISBN 978 1 84445 842 4
Medicines Management in Children's Nursing	ISBN 978 1 84445 470 9
Medicines Management in Mental Health Nursing	ISBN 978 0 85725 049 0
Mental Health Law in Nursing	ISBN 978 0 85725 863 2
Nursing Adults with Long Term Conditions	ISBN 978 0 85725 441 2
Nursing and Collaborative Practice (2nd edn)	ISBN 978 1 84445 373 3
Nursing and Mental Health Care	ISBN 978 1 84445 467 9
Passing Calculations Tests for Nursing Students (2nd edn)	ISBN 978 1 44625 624 8
Patient and Carer Participation in Nursing	ISBN 978 0 85725 307 1
Patient Assessment and Care Planning in Nursing	ISBN 978 0 85725 858 8
Psychology and Sociology in Nursing	ISBN 978 0 85725 836 6
Safeguarding Adults in Nursing Practice	ISBN 978 1 44625 638 1
Successful Practice Learning for Nursing Students (2nd edn)	ISBN 978 0 85725 315 6
Using Health Policy in Nursing Practice	ISBN 978 1 44625 646 6
What is Nursing? Exploring Theory and Practice (3rd edn)	ISBN 978 0 85725 975 2

Personal and professional learning skills titles:

Series editors: Dr Mooi Standing, Independent Academic Consultant (UK and International) and Accredited NMC Reviewer and Professor Shirley Bach, Head of the School of Nursing and Midwifery at the University of Brighton

Clinical Judgement and Decision Making in Nursing	ISBN 978 1 84445 468 6
Critical Thinking and Writing for Nursing Students (2nd edn)	ISBN 978 1 44625 644 2
Evidence-based Practice in Nursing (2nd edn)	ISBN 978 1 44627 090 5
Information Skills for Nursing Students	ISBN 978 1 84445 381 8
Reflective Practice in Nursing (2nd edn)	ISBN 978 1 44627 085 1
Succeeding in Essays, Exams and OSCEs for Nursing Students	ISBN 978 0 85725 827 4
Succeeding in Research Project Plans and Literature Reviews for Nursing Students	ISBN 978 0 85725 264 7
Successful Professional Portfolios for Nursing Students	ISBN 978 0 85725 457 3
Understanding Research for Nursing Students (2nd edn)	ISBN 978 1 44626 761 5

You can find more information on each of these titles and our other learning resources at **www.sagepub.co.uk**. Many of these titles are also available in various e-book formats; please visit our website for more information.

Reflective Practice in Nursing

Second edition

Lioba Howatson-Jones

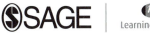

Los Angeles | London | New Delhi
Singapore | Washington DC

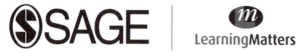
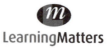

Learning Matters
An imprint of SAGE Publications Ltd
1 Oliver's Yard
55 City Road
London EC1Y 1SP

SAGE Publications Inc.
2455 Teller Road
Thousand Oaks, California 91320

SAGE Publications India Pvt Ltd
B 1/I 1 Mohan Cooperative Industrial Area
Mathura Road
New Delhi 110 044

SAGE Publications Asia-Pacific Pte Ltd
3 Church Street
#10-04 Samsung Hub
Singapore 049483

Editor: Alex Clabburn
Development editor: Richenda Milton-Daws
Production controller: Chris Marke
Project management: Diana Chambers
Marketing manager: Tamara Navaratnam
Cover design: Wendy Scott
Typeset by: Kelly Winter
Printed by: MPG Printgroup, UK

First published 2010
Second edition published 2013

Library of Congress Control Number: 2013930255

British Library Cataloguing in Publication data
A catalogue record for this book is available from
the British Library

ISBN 978 1 44627 084 4
ISBN 978 1 44627 085 1 (pbk)

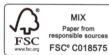

MIX
Paper from
responsible sources
FSC
www.fsc.org   FSC® C018575

Contents

Foreword

The *Transforming Nursing Practice* series includes several titles that focus on personal and professional learning skills, and *Reflective Practice in Nursing* is a great example in this respect. Lifelong learning in nursing involves a constant dialogue between nurses' personal inner world and the outer world of scientific or technological knowledge and NMC standards that they must somehow incorporate in their understanding, identity and practice as nurses. This book carefully and skilfully shows the reader how to do this through reflective practice. High-quality care combines personal (human sensitivity regarding patients' experience) and professional (relevant, well-thought out, skilled interventions) aspects of nursing. Each chapter is loaded with interesting practical examples, case studies and activities to engage readers in reflecting on and developing self-awareness, problem-solving skills and nursing knowledge that is grounded in interactions with service users. After reading this book, nursing students and others will be well informed in applying principles of reflective practice to review their actions and enhance their professional development.

The second edition of this popular book has retained its central theme but has been comprehensively updated by taking on board the feedback received. In addition to addressing new developments in this subject area, it updates references where necessary and reformats material to stimulate readers' interest. In doing so, Lioba Howatson-Jones has made the book more accessible, relevant and applicable to the different nursing pathways using a wider range of settings for new case studies and scenarios. Lioba has also recognised the book's appeal to qualified nurses by providing them with alternative activities that acknowledge their experience and expertise. A new chapter on the use of new media for reflecting on nursing experiences is a welcome addition and gives the book a contemporary feel by relating developments in digital communication to reflective practice.

Dr Mooi Standing
Series Editor

About the author

Dr Lioba Howatson-Jones is Senior Lecturer in Nursing and Applied Clinical Studies at Canterbury Christ Church University, where she teaches on pre-registration, post-registration and Masters level courses. Lioba's clinical nursing background is mainly in acute nursing and practice development. She has taught at the University since 2003 and has a particular interest in clinical supervision. Her research interests are in exploring nurses' learning and academic development. Lioba has published on these and clinical topics since 1999.

Acknowledgements

This book is based on 30 years' nursing experience and draws from that experience, as well as teaching and research. Therefore, I would like to acknowledge the contributions of patients, colleagues and students – past and present – to my learning and the development of some of the ideas. In particular, I thank the participants in my PhD research who have contributed much to my articulation of reflective learning.

I also thank Professor Linden West for introducing me to biographical approaches to lifelong learning, and psychodynamic ideas of transitional space. Martin Bedford, my clinical supervisor, guided reflections on my own learning from which some of the material is drawn. I can truly say that this learning is always an adventure.

Thanks go to Dr Mooi Standing for some helpful suggestions in the editing of the chapters. I would also like to thank the editors at Sage.

Finally, I wish to thank my husband for once again supporting my 'time out' to complete the writing. Thanks also to my sister Elke for useful discussions about different approaches to reflection in the health professions.

Use of previously published work

The author and publisher would like to thank the following for permission to reproduce copyright material:

Gibbs, G (1988) *Learning by Doing: A guide to teaching and learning methods*. Oxford: Further Education Unit, p47.

Adapted Figure 4.1, p59, Gibbs' (1998) reflective cycle. Used with the kind permission of OCSLD, Oxford Brookes University.

Johns, C (2004) *Becoming a Reflective Practitioner*, 2nd edition. Oxford: Blackwell Publishing, pp20–7.

Box on MSR reflective cues, pp54–5. Adapted from Johns' Model for Structured Reflection. Reproduced with permission of Blackwell Publishing Ltd, © 2004 Blackwell Publishing Ltd.

Palmer, A, Burns, S, and Bulman, C (1994) *Reflective Practice in Nursing: The growth of the Professional Practitioner*. Oxford: Blackwell Scientific Publications, p137.

Box on Stephenson's model of reflection from a student's perspective, p57. Reproduced with permission of Blackwell Publishing Ltd, © 1994 Blackwell Scientific Publications.

Atkins, S and Murphy, K (1995) Reflective Practice. *Nursing Standard*, 9 (45): 31–7.

Stages of Reflection, p56, reproduced with kind permission of the RCN Publishing Company Ltd.

Van Ooijen, E (2003) *Clinical Supervision Made Easy*. Edinburgh: Churchill Livingstone, p21.

Figure 8.1, Developmental framework, p112. This figure was adapted from the original, copyright © Elsevier, used with kind permission.

Every effort has been made to trace all copyright holders within the book, but if any have been inadvertently overlooked the publisher will be pleased to make the necessary arrangements at the first opportunity.

Guide to the companion website accompanying this book

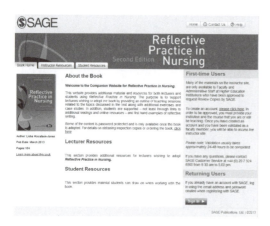

The companion website that accompanies this book provides students and lecturers with ready-to-use teaching and learning resources. They are free of charge and are designed to maximise the learning experience.

 www.sagepub.co.uk/
howatson-jones_reflective2e

For lecturers

Password protected material to ensure that only lecturers can access these resources. Registration is easy: just click on 'Lecturer Material' and if you have adopted the book, simply request a user-name and password from the email address supplied and access will be granted.

Extra activities and case studies

The author has provided some fantastic activities within the book which help to cement learning and encourage deeper understanding. We have taken this further by making extra materials available to provide a wider range of activities and case studies. These are downloadable and can be integrated into your VLE.

For students

Further reading and weblinks

There is a huge amount of information about reflective practice available on the internet and knowing where to start is not easy. The author has helped by providing a manageable list of some useful websites that you would be wise to look at.

Example of extended reflective writing

Sometimes the best way to understand something is to look at examples of how others have approached it and the author here supplies further examples of reflective writing for you to look at.

Introduction

This book provides a method for developing analytical skills through different ways of using personal and professional **reflection** for learning and developing as a practitioner. The purpose of the book is to introduce the novice and more experienced practitioner to a number of models and frameworks for reflection, as well as ways of integrating personal and professional reflective insights. The aim is to assist you to develop a sense of **agency** in your own learning by broadening the scope and depth of your reflection to include biographical aspects. The reason for this is to help you to develop a lifewide (as well as a lifelong) view of learning and reflection, which can sustain your practice and you as a practitioner.

This book should be viewed as offering practical guidance to becoming reflective. It will be particularly useful for those starting out on such a process, or wanting to try different methods. As you and your reflection develop, so too will your interest and reading to include ever more complex concepts and professional experience. The following chapters will encourage you to examine your experience and learning within the reflective process – through case studies, scenarios and activities that are rooted in the realities of practice and learning. This will help you to cope with the uncertainty of developing as a professional in a constructive way.

Chapter 1 sets the scene, showing how reflection has come about and its relevance for the new student and developing practitioner. It identifies some potential benefits for the person, profession, patients/clients, organisation and society that reflection can bring. It is important for the novice and experienced practitioner to recognise the significance of reflection for effective practice and development of professional knowledge, particularly the fundamentals of practice.

Chapter 2 emphasises that learning does not only take place through formal courses or instruction, but extends into all areas of life. This chapter invites you to review some of these areas reflectively in order to extend learning potential. The focus here is on the types of knowledge produced through this reflective process, and the ways of knowing that can develop, which are crucial to lifelong learning.

Chapter 3 introduces the student and developing practitioner to autobiographical reflection as a means of helping to advance nursing knowledge in more diverse ways. In this chapter you are invited to integrate autobiographical reflection and learning with a sense of your developing identity as well as to reflect on aspects of life that may also be revealing of societal issues.

Chapter 4 introduces some of the wide range of reflective models and frameworks that the student and practitioner can draw upon when first starting to structure and frame their reflections. The chapter also considers the strengths and limitations of these, to help you to choose appropriately.

Chapter 5 introduces the student and developing practitioner to concepts of reflection as a transitional space in which you are encouraged to explore, develop and grow. As you progress, more will be expected in terms of knowledge, skills and decision making. How a transitional space can draw out reflection and learning is a particular focus here.

Chapter 6 examines how student nurses and developing practitioners can influence their experiences, and how those experiences might influence them. It focuses on the role of reflexivity in developing opportunities for learning.

Chapter 7 invites you to cultivate a reflective approach to daily experience, and integrate what you are learning. It is important for students to be able to acknowledge limitations within their knowledge as well as to own potential mistakes, and this chapter focuses on how to respond to fallibility – in oneself and in other professionals.

Chapter 8 considers how guided reflection, and reflecting with others, can deepen your understanding and analysis of situations, experiences and decisions, and offer support. The chapter also introduces ways of dealing with emotional residues of caring work.

Chapter 9 explores the purpose of reflective writing and introduces the student to a variety of techniques. You are encouraged to try out some different exercises to help develop this skill. Some examples of reflective writing are discussed.

Chapter 10 looks at the possibilities new media offer for reflecting with others. It explores potential benefits and pitfalls, and identifies how to develop your own digital story on which to reflect.

Chapter 11 emphasises the intense nature of critical reflection and its relevance to developing the skill of criticality. You are encouraged to consider your personal contributions and those of others to the development and outcomes of experiences.

NMC *Standards for Pre-registration Nursing Education* and Essential Skills Clusters

The Nursing and Midwifery Council (NMC) has standards of competence that have to be met by applicants to different parts of the nursing and midwifery register. These standards are what they deem as being necessary for the delivery of safe, effective nursing and midwifery practice.

As well as specific competencies, the NMC identifies specific skills that nursing students must have at various points of their training programme. These Essential Skills Clusters (ESCs) are essential abilities that students need to attain in order to practise to their full potential.

This book includes the latest standards for 2010 onwards, taken from *Standards for Pre-registration Nursing Education* (NMC, 2010a). For links to the pre-2010 standards, please visit the website for the book at www.learningmatters.co.uk/nursing.

Learning features

Learning from reading text is not always easy. Therefore, to provide variety and to assist with the development of independent learning skills and the application of theory to practice, this book contains activities, example stories, scenarios (some with questions), case studies, concept summaries, further reading and useful websites to enable you to participate in your own learning. You will need to develop your own study skills and 'learn how to learn' to get the best from the material. The book cannot provide all the answers – but instead provides a framework for your learning.

The activities in the book will help you in particular to make sense of, and learn about, the material being presented. Some activities ask you to reflect on aspects of practice, or your experience of it, or the people or situations you encounter. *Reflection* is an essential skill in nursing, and it helps you to understand the world around you and often to identify how things might be improved. Other activities will help you develop key graduate skills such as your ability to *think critically* about a topic in order to challenge received wisdom, or your ability to *research a topic and find appropriate information and evidence*, and to be able to make decisions using that evidence in situations that are often difficult and time-pressured. Communication and working as part of a team are core to all nursing practice, and some activities will ask you to think about your *communication skills* to help develop these.

All the activities require you to take a break from reading the text, think through the issues presented and carry out some independent study, possibly using the internet. Where appropriate, there are sample answers presented at the end of each chapter, and these will help you to understand more fully your own reflections and independent study. You will gain most from the activities if you try to complete them yourself before reading the suggested answers. Remember, academic study will always require independent work; attending lectures will never be enough to be successful on your programme, and these activities will help to deepen your knowledge and understanding of the issues under scrutiny and give you practice at working on your own.

You might want to think about completing these activities as part of your personal development plan (PDP) or portfolio. After completing the activity, write it up in your PDP or portfolio in a section devoted to that particular skill, then look back over time to see how far you have developed. You can also do more of the activities for a key skill that you have identified a weakness in, which will help build your skill and confidence in this area.

There is a glossary of terms at the end of the book that provides an interpretation of some of the terminology in the context of the subject of the book. Glossary terms are in **bold** in the first instance that they appear.

All chapters have further reading and useful websites listed at the end, with notes to show you why we think they will be helpful to you. The websites will also help you to remain up to date with developments in this aspect of practice as awareness of key issues grows and policies develop.

We hope that you find this book helpful in developing your professional practice and that it challenges you to ensure you provide care and support that reduces the risk of vulnerability, and promotes dignity, respect and a positive quality of life. Good luck with your studies!

Chapter 1
What is meant by reflection and reflective practice

continued . . .

By the first progression point:

1. Works within the code (NMC 2008) and adheres to the *Guidance on professional conduct for nursing and midwifery students.* (NMC 2010)

By the second progression point:

4. Reflects on own practice and discusses issues with other members of the team to enhance learning.

Chapter aims

After reading this chapter you will be able to:

- define reflection and reflective practice;
- understand the relevance of reflection in nursing;
- identify benefits for the person, profession, patients/clients, organisation and society;
- understand the nature of accountability and reflection;
- begin to explore personal and professional forms of reflection.

Example story

Andy had always wanted to be a community nurse. He was currently in the second year of his nurse preparation programme and on a placement working with the community team. Andy and his mentor were called to visit a lady who was dying at home. Her pressure mattress was not working properly and they needed to replace it as the motor unit seemed to be faulty. When the mattress was replaced, Andy set the motor settings while his mentor settled the patient, as she had become rather distressed by all the upheaval.

The following day they were called back as the patient had had a difficult night. She complained of severe discomfort and that the mattress was very hard. On checking her pressure areas they noted that her sacrum was pink. When Andy checked the motor unit he saw that it was on a high setting. His mentor suggested that perhaps he had set it on the wrong setting. They apologised to the patient and reset it. His mentor decided they would check again later in the day.

Andy and his mentor reflected briefly in the car on the way back to their base. Andy's mentor realised she should have checked the settings before they left. She was accountable for their actions, although Andy was responsible for identifying whether he had the necessary knowledge for the task requested of him. They agreed that, in future, Andy would ask if he was unsure and that his mentor would also check.

When reflecting on his own, Andy realised that the reason he had not asked was because he thought that, as a second-year student nurse, he ought to have known what the settings should be and did not want to look silly by asking. When thinking about the situation now he understood that, by not asking, he was partly responsible for having put the patient at risk. He decided that, in future, he would make sure that he told his mentor honestly what his knowledge and deficits were in order to be able to learn and develop. The example of his mentor highlighting that she had not checked the settings enabled him to realise that professionals are also fallible and need to constantly review their practice, as well as learn from it.

Introduction

Professionals are sometimes fallible and the example above is offered as an illustration of the importance of reflection in helping to make sense of things. When reading the example, a number of thoughts may have been going through your mind: 'Why did the student nurse not ask?'; 'Why did the mentor not check?'; 'What might perhaps have been done differently?' Reflection may not be a familiar concept to you, particularly when starting your nurse preparation programme. So this chapter begins by setting the scene of what reflection is and its relevance for the new student as well as the more experienced practitioner. It contextualises reflection and **reflective practice** through tracing some of the main historical roots and key developments in order to help establish its importance. The chapter further emphasises the significance of reflection for effective practice and development of professional knowledge. The chapter concludes by considering accountability issues and the relationship to professional and personal forms of reflection. You will be invited throughout the chapter to complete a variety of activities and consider a number of case studies and scenarios. This will help you to start reflecting if you are a novice, or to develop reflection if you are a more experienced practitioner.

What is reflection?

Reflection has been defined variously as accessing previous experience helping to develop **tacit** and **intuitive knowledge** (Johns and Freshwater, 2005), a transformative process that changes individuals and their actions (Ghaye and Lillyman, 2010) and a way to reach awareness of how and why things have occurred (Johns, 2010). 'Tacit knowledge' is about having a common understanding about something and 'intuitive' means being sensitive to links with previous experience. Reflection is a way of examining your experience in order to look for the possibility of other explanations and alternative approaches to doing things. It may happen as part of activity or when you have more time to think about what you have experienced. What is required is an open and enquiring mind that can accept the possibility of a number of different explanations. Reflection is not unusual. We do it in the car, on the train, cooking a meal, while undertaking exercise, in the bath and during and after conversations, basically wherever we can find mental and physical space to take a moment to think about things. Take a little time out now to think about what you did today and complete Activity 1.1.

Activity 1.1	*Reflection*

Spend a little time reviewing what you have done today.

- What particular aspects were significant and why?
- When and where did you find yourself thinking about something in more depth?
- Can you track changes to your thinking?
- What do you think about the issue now?

There is an outline answer to this activity at the end of the chapter.

When completing the activity you may have identified another way that you would have liked to have done things, or other things you might have liked to have said, and may have arrived at a different conclusion. Reflection means that thoughts of significant aspects of an experience are reconsidered and other explanations are contemplated. For the more experienced practitioner, reflection may reach greater depth as there is more knowledge and a wider range of experience to examine. For example, reflection may be triggered by a different response to a routine action and proceed beyond the immediate situation to consider knowledge, personal values and personal practice as well as the values and practice of others. Sometimes, other explanations might need to be imagined – particularly for the inexperienced practitioner – and confirmed with someone more experienced. It is important to separate fantasy (what you might like to happen) from the reality of what is possible or likely; for example, imagining the potential reaction of a client or patient, or considering possible consequences of a particular act. The scenario below is provided to help you to gain further understanding of the role of imagination in reflection. You are asked to identify some of these features after reading the scenario.

Scenario: Lynn's experience of using imagination as a novice practitioner

Lynn had been working with a care assistant in her first placement of her nurse preparation programme. Her placement was in a nursing home and she did not like it very much because she found the work very repetitive. On this particular day she had had an argument with the care assistant about the method used for lifting a patient. The care assistant had wanted to lift the lady with an underarm lift. Lynn had pointed out that this was not the way she had been taught on her course and that they should use the lifting aids available. The care assistant had become very angry with her and told her that she was not in charge here. Later, Lynn saw the care assistant talking to some others and imagined they were talking about her. She was worried that her assessment, which was due that day, might be compromised. To calm her nerves, Lynn tried to think things through.

The care assistant had been in a hurry. Lynn's priority was to do what she thought was best for the patient. Lynn had never seen a pressure sore but she thought that, had they dragged the patient up the bed, her skin would have been pulled. She imagined what the consequences might have been. The lady was quite frail and thin and her skin might have broken, or at the very least become irritated by being dragged over the sheet. Lynn continued . . .

felt more confident that she had done the right thing by protecting the patient from this consequence. She thought about her imminent assessment and what to say to the qualified nurse. She was sure that she would say something about it and that she would be in trouble.

The qualified nurse did come and speak to Lynn, but not in the way that Lynn had imagined. She asked her about her problem solving within the situation. She then confirmed that Lynn's action had been correct and that her imagining of the potential consequences for the patient was also correct. Lynn felt that she had gained confidence in being able to think things through. She also understood that there was a difference between imagining feelings and potential consequences. Feelings are subjective and contextual and therefore also harder to anticipate, while the potential consequences of actions could be anticipated by thinking about them using knowledge.

Questions

- What are the significant features in this scenario and why?
- If you are an experienced nurse, how might your reflective imagination have differed from Lynn's?

There are outline answers to these questions at the end of the chapter.

Having read the scenario and answered the questions at the end, you will be able to see that reflection using imagination can review a number of different strands of a situation and how this might be relevant to practice. We will return to the role of imagination in reflection in Chapter 3. The scenario also illustrates the importance of reflecting on events and discussing them with others in order to clarify perceptions and safe practice.

The chapter now proceeds to define what reflective practice is.

What is reflective practice?

Reflective practice has been defined as a process that develops understanding of what it means to be a practitioner (Rolfe, 2011) and makes the link between theory and practice through the practitioner consciously thinking through the experience (Jasper, 2003). This is important for the novice practitioner to help develop an understanding of their role and support the learning of new skills. To do so, reflection can occur within the experience or by looking back at the experience. Schön (1991) identifies these as reflection-in-action and reflection-on-action. Theory needs to be mapped on to situational features in order to use it for problem solving. Thinking about things requires knowledge of theory in order to develop answers. Reflection-in-action refers to knowing what to do and making a difference within a given situation. Reflection-on-action means examining some of those 'in the moment' decisions for the possibility of other choices and ways of acting, and how these insights might shape and develop future practice.

Problem solving can take the form of rational thinking based on protocols and procedures. However, simply imitating role-modelled behaviour in dealing with situations is a form of nonreflective learning (Jarvis, 2006). For example, when undertaking a drug round, if the practitioner is mainly intent on fulfilling the requirements of the five rights of drug administration through checking the right dose, right drug, right patient, right time and right route, and does not reflectively consider their actions, knowledge or the patient, this does not itself develop learning. What aids learning is looking beyond the basic actions to examine understanding and personal responses. Reflective practice requires careful consideration of knowledge and ideas.

Reflective practice considers practice as a holistic entity that cannot always be rationalised. Individuals are unique, and human factors may be uncertain, even messy. Reflective practice, therefore, is based on experience and intuitive learning that you may not be aware of until you have to respond to a situation. This may be easier for practitioners with greater experience upon which to draw. Nevertheless, capturing such learning by bringing it into awareness through reflecting on practice is an important part of developing understanding, skill and competence as a practitioner at any stage. This is especially true when the ideal does not match the reality of the situation – what Argyris and Schön (1978) call *espoused theories versus theories in use*. Espoused theories are enshrined within protocols and procedures of how practice should proceed. The theories in use are those that have developed from application and reflection, and that are being considered 'in action'. In this way reflective practice can contribute to organisational learning through its members.

Knowledge derived from practice does not add to professional knowledge unless it has been reflected on for its significance (Eraut, 2001). For example, as a novice practitioner you may have worked with healthcare assistants and your qualified mentor. You may have observed and been involved in completing a care element, such as a bed bath, with both at some point. You may even have been aware of some differences between them in how the care was completed. However, unless you reflect on this and reach some conclusions about the significance of the differences, the care will remain a task that was completed in different ways, and not perhaps the expression of nursing knowledge that it might have been. The learning embedded within this will be lost. Equally, an experienced practitioner who may have to complete similar tasks can gain greater insight and knowledge through reflecting on how the tasks themselves might be the same and yet different each time they are performed and what knowledge is being used and maybe even generated, in order to avoid simple repetition of experience that does not constitute learning.

Now apply some of the principles of reflective practice to your own practice by completing Activity 1.2.

Activity 1.2   *Critical thinking*

When you are next in practice and in a nursing situation, try to consider the following.

- What is going on?
- What knowledge are you using?
- What decisions are you making?
- How have you come to those decisions?
- Are you trying out different things?
- What is changing your thinking, if anything?

continued . . .

Allow an interval of at least a day between the situation and reflecting on it further. Now ask yourself the same questions again.

- Have your answers changed and if so how?
- What learning are you taking forward from this?

It is useful to keep asking yourself these questions and to maintain a reflective diary to track your learning and development.

It might help to document this activity by using the pro forma offered at the end of the chapter.

As this activity is based on your own experiences, there is no outline answer at the end of the chapter.

Chapter 7 will pick up the theme of reflective practice again by looking at what constitutes the reflective practitioner. Having defined what reflection and reflective practice are, this chapter now proceeds to take a brief look at the development of reflection and its relevance in the context of nursing.

History and development of reflection in the context of nursing

It might be surmised that early pioneers of nursing (such as Florence Nightingale) potentially came to different conclusions of what was needed in terms of sanitation in hospitals, through possibly reflecting on the problem. What is clearer is that the possibilities for reflection begin to appear in nursing through research studies that explore different types of nursing knowledge. For example, Carper (1978) identified patterns of knowing that looked further than a medical model of disease management to where nurses discovered new nursing theories through working out their ideas. Benner's (1984) seminal work started to explain how nurses developed their knowledge in practice, and Watson (1985, 1988) recognised the importance of previous practice in shaping nurses' perceptions of knowledge and urged that nurses also needed to develop new insights. Schön (1991) suggested reflection as getting to the heart of how professionals think in action.

Changes in nurses' basic preparation has meant that there has been an increasing focus on reflection as a tool for teaching and learning. Since the early 1990s, interest in reflection as a concept and its contribution within nurse education has grown (Pierson, 1998). In 1994, the United Kingdom Central Council (UKCC), nursing's regulatory body at the time, pronounced that all nurses needed to maintain a portfolio of evidence of learning activity and listed reflection as an essential component of this activity. This requirement has been updated by the NMC (2008), which makes it clear that reflection on the outcome of any type of learning is essential to maintaining knowledge, skills and competence as a nurse. Thus reflection, in the context of nursing, is now a foundation for learning that can take place both inside and outside the classroom.

The discourse between the novice and experienced practitioner is part of an ongoing reflective dialogue that continues to take nursing practice forward through the new insights that are revealed within such discussions (Johns, 2010). Thus the student nurse and the experienced mentor can contribute to nursing knowledge in dynamic ways through interaction. For example, by questioning and exploring what is known about a situation or topic, what is unknown is also brought into the picture and can be given consideration to develop wider understanding. This is an important part of developing the profession. This is given definition by reading the case study of some dialogue between a student and a mentor.

Case study: Student and mentor dialogue

Student: *I have never come across anyone with a learning disability. How do I talk to them?*

Mentor: *How do you like to be talked to?*

Student: *I like people to use my first name and for us to share our views on the topic of conversation.*

Mentor: *That is a good way to talk to someone. Ask them to tell you a bit about themselves and share their views. What have you learned about communication in your preparation programme?*

Student: *We have learned about how to build therapeutic relationships and using verbal and non-verbal communication. But I am not sure how they might respond.*

Mentor: *We don't know how anyone might respond and have to take our cues from them. What is your main concern?*

Student: *That I might upset them and not know what to do.*

Mentor: *One way of avoiding this is to learn to read emotional cues. If you attune yourself to others' emotional cues you can start to work out how they are feeling and responding to what you are saying. When I started nursing I found it hard to talk to people because I was very shy. I still am shy, but what has helped me is learning to move beyond my own feelings by becoming aware of others' emotional feelings, and responding accordingly. This is part of emotional intelligence.*

Student: *I think we had a lecture about emotional intelligence.*

Mentor: *Start talking to one of our residents today by finding out a bit about each other. Then revisit your notes from that lecture and reflect on what you have learned today. We will discuss your reflection about this tomorrow.*

The case study of student and mentor dialogue has illustrated how thinking about and reflecting on practice issues is an important way for professional knowledge to develop. 'Socratic questioning', which asks for thinking, is an essential part of this learning process. The idea of developing understanding and knowledge of nursing through reflection brings benefits for the nurse and patient. Some of these benefits are explored in the next section of the chapter, which looks at the benefits of reflection.

Benefits of reflection

Reflection can help to affirm as well as to correct actions. In doing so it may enable you to translate successful strategies into new situations and thus continue to develop them. Equally, when reflection reveals problems with an action taken, this will enable you to avoid using that action in similar circumstances again, or allow you to consider other corrections. From such a perspective reflection can help to raise your confidence in your developing abilities and of things to avoid. Some benefits from reflection for the individual practitioner, the organisation and the patient are summarised in Figure 1.1.

Reflection means making the familiar unfamiliar, or looking at it with fresh eyes (Abrandt Dahlgren et al., 2004). You will be able to chart the development of your effectiveness in problem solving and delivery of patient care by using reflection during your nursing preparation programme. Equally, if you are an experienced practitioner, reflection will help you to re-evaluate your personal effectiveness in problem solving and the management of patient care. Through the improving skills of the individual, the organisation as a whole benefits, as do the clients and patients for whom the organisation offers a service. Thus reflection as practised by you could also reflect across the profession throughout your lifetime as a nurse. By completing Activity 1.3, you will be able to consider in more detail some of the benefits reflection might have for you.

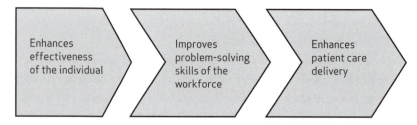

Figure 1.1: Benefits of reflection to the individual, organisation and patient

---

Activity 1.3   *Reflection*

As a student nurse you will need to learn clinical skills. Think about the first skill you learnt.

*   What were the highlights of learning this skill?
*   What were the problems?
*   How did you deal with any existing or potential problems?
*   How did you feel about learning the skill at the time?
*   How did you feel about putting it into practice with a real person for the first time?
*   Did your practice change in the live setting and, if so, why?
*   What do you think about your practice of the skill now after reflecting on it through these questions?
*   What learning are you taking forward from this?

If you are an experienced practitioner consider the same questions in relation to decision-making and management skills.

There is an outline answer to this activity at the end of the chapter.

Having identified your learning of the skill through the activity and your evaluation of it now will give you a clearer picture of your knowledge and ability. These are important aspects of your personal responsibility and accountability. We now move on to consider how accountability relates to reflection.

Accountability and reflection

The professional code of conduct for nurses and midwives expects nurses to maintain their knowledge in order to provide safe and effective practice (NMC, 2008). Working within the boundaries of the code is a part of the standard of professional values expected of nurses and of nursing practice. As has already been suggested, simply receiving new ideas does not translate into becoming knowledgeable. Reflection is needed to develop new concepts into understanding them. Therefore, if as a nurse you are expected to maintain your knowledge, it follows that thinking and reflecting on that knowledge and what you do is part of your accountability as a nurse. The following scenarios look at Mandy's responsibility and Sarah's accountability as a way of illustrating the process of reflecting on these aspects within learning from practice. After reading the first scenario you are asked to identify what aspects you might need to reflect on and what your response might be.

Scenario: Mandy's responsibility

Mandy was in the second year of her nurse preparation programme. She had been working in a day surgery unit. The day surgery unit encompassed a pre-assessment area, ward and theatre suite, with the ward phone as the central contact point. The unit was busy with people coming and going, and the phone ringing with relatives enquiring whether patients were ready to come home, or doctors asking for information. In one such phone call a doctor asked Mandy to pass a message to the theatre staff about a certain instrument that was needed to be available for the afternoon theatre list. Unfortunately, Mandy was distracted by a patient who started vomiting and needed her assistance, and she forgot to pass the message on.

When the afternoon began, a very angry nurse rang from the theatre suite to ask why the message about the specialised instrument had not been passed on. The patient's procedure had to be cancelled because the necessary instrument could not be prepared in time.

The doctor came to apologise to the patient who was not very happy. The theatre staff were upset that they appeared inefficient. The ward manager wanted to know who had taken the message and not passed it on. Mandy was also upset when she realised it was her and thought what to do next.

Question
- If you were Mandy, what would you think about, what would you reflect on and what would be your response?

There is an outline answer to this question at the end of the chapter.

Now consider another day in Mandy's placement, again on the same unit. After reading the second scenario, you are asked to identify what aspects you might need to reflect on and what your learning might be.

Scenario: Whose accountability?

Mandy was working another shift on day surgery with her mentor, Sarah. It was a Friday and the patients who had recovered from their procedures were eager to go home. Mandy was preparing one lady, who had undergone a **haemorrhoidectomy***, to go home. Haemorrhoidectomy can be quite a painful procedure and she was being sent home with some prescribed* **analgesia***. The form of this analgesia was contraindicated for use by people who had asthma as it could induce an asthmatic episode. As Mandy was checking the medication and talking to the patient, she realised that the lady did have a history of asthma, although she did not take regular medication for it, only rarely needing to use an inhaler. Nevertheless, Mandy brought this to the attention of her mentor, explaining that the drug had been prescribed and what she had found out about its contraindications. She reflected on what might have happened if she had not noticed. Would she have been responsible as in the previous episode? Who was accountable if the lady did subsequently suffer an asthmatic attack at home?*

Questions
- If you were Mandy, what would you reflect on in this situation?
- If you were Sarah, what would you reflect on in this situation? (If you are a novice practitioner, leave this part of the question.)
- How are responsibility and accountability assigned in this scenario?
- What might Mandy have learned from this situation?
- What might Sarah have learned from this situation? (If you are a novice practitioner, leave this part of the question.)

There are outline answers to these questions at the end of the chapter.

These scenarios have helped to give you a clearer idea of some of the differences between responsibility and accountability, and the role of reflection in helping to make sense of this. This is especially important when undertaking your nurse preparation programme, as it can sometimes appear less clear in practice. Equally, as an experienced practitioner, reflecting on near-miss situations is important for adjusting practice. The chapter now proceeds to look at some personal and professional forms of reflection that can help with this.

Personal and professional forms of reflection

Journal writing is one method that has been used to develop reflective learning (Chirema, 2007). The private log, or blog, has become increasingly popular as a way of working out what has personally been learned. This is usually kept private and only enters the public domain when shared with a tutor through a progress review, or to inform assignment content when on a nurse preparation programme, as it forms part of the portfolio of evidence of learning. As technology has developed, the student on a nurse preparation programme may be asked to enter reflections on learning into a **wiki**, with different pages assigned to different aspects of their programme. The tutor only has access to view the wiki when this is shared by the student. The issue of using digital media for reflection will be explored in more detail in Chapter 10. During your preparation programme you will perhaps have been asked to reflect on a variety of situations and scenarios similar to what this book is asking you to do. You may also be asked to reflect in your assignments in the form of case studies, where you might include a review of your actions and contribution to the patient's care. Complete Activity 1.4 as a way of starting to think about recording your reflective learning. The issue of reflective writing will be explored in more detail in Chapter 9.

Activity 1.4 *Reflection*

Think about the main elements of your preparation programme. Write a reflection on your progress in each of these areas.

If you are an experienced practitioner, think about the main elements of your career development and write a reflection on your progress.

There is an outline answer to this activity at the end of the chapter.

For the experienced practitioner reflection involves thinking about the nursing identity and reconstructing experience in order to identify how to progress (Lindsay, 2006). This type of reflection examines aspects such as: *self-respect, hope, control, vulnerability, acceptance, loss and persistence* (Daley, 2001, p53).

For example, nursing someone who is dying may call into question our own mortality. Reconstructing the experience by looking at how we deal with loss might offer a way into examining how loss is interpreted in the context of dying and others' experience. This may stimulate reflective thinking about possible courses of action for helping others to face loss. Reflective writing may be entered into a private diary and considered privately during such 'working out'. Professional forms of reflection may take place individually or in a group through a variety of ways such as clinical supervision or action learning. These forms of reflecting with others will be explored in greater detail in Chapter 8.

Chapter summary

This chapter has begun to define what reflection and reflective practice are. By offering activities that ask the novice and developing nurse to review thinking and practice, the chapter has provided an opportunity for starting to develop reflection in relation to safe and effective nursing practice and decision making. Through inclusion of examples that help to illustrate the benefits of reflection, and the relationship between accountability and reflection, you are encouraged to start thinking about how this might be relevant to your learning and practice, as well as to working within a regulatory code. Different forms of reflection and reflective practice will be explained further in later chapters.

Activities and scenarios: Brief outline answers

Activity 1.1: Reflection (page 7)

Your answer might have considered:

- getting up;
- interaction with others at home;
- travelling to work;
- priorities for work;
- completing work;
- coming home.

When thinking about which aspects were significant and why, you might have first been alerted by triggered emotions, for example anxiety, satisfaction or anger, which led you to consider the trigger, which might have been a decision that you had made or were finding difficult to make. From here you can then re-evaluate the situation.

Activity 1.3: Reflection (page 12)

You might have thought about nursing skills such as taking a pulse and blood pressure. You might have considered the difficulty of hearing the blood pressure when taking a manual measurement and of being nervous when faced with a real patient. As your skill has developed you may have identified some more subtle nuances, such as slight variation in where the brachial artery might be located in different patients. You might have learned that a manual measurement is sometimes more accurate than an electronic one when blood pressure is significantly abnormal.

As an experienced practitioner you might have thought about decision making in relation to problem solving, planning and implementing care. As your skill has developed you may have identified that you are able to do this quickly while dealing with competing demands. You might have considered management skills such as allocating the skill mix of staff and liaising with the hierarchy of management. You might have learned the strengths and weaknesses of your interpersonal skills and management strategies.

Activity 1.4: Reflection (page 15)

You might have written reflections on:

- developing graduate skills;
- knowledge and proficiency with information technology;
- developing essential clinical skills;
- practice;
- personal development planning.

You might have written reflections on:

- developing leadership and management skills;
- developing your knowledge and proficiency in different practice situations;
- dealing with conflict and change.

Scenario: Lynn's experience of using imagination as a novice practitioner (pages 7–8)

The significant features in this scenario that Lynn is likely to have reflected on are:

- the conflict with practice;
- the argument with the care assistant;
- her own practice.

She used imagination to consider aspects where she did not have knowledge, namely:

- how others viewed her abilities;
- the effect of friction on the skin;
- the consequences of her decisions.

As an experienced nurse your reflective imagination might have differed from Lynn's by identifying the significant features as:

- your accountability in this situation;
- how to rectify the manual handling knowledge of the staff in the setting.

You might have used imagination to consider the aspects you did not have knowledge of, such as:

- how others might react to change;
- how to overcome barriers to change.

Scenario: Mandy's responsibility (page 13)

In this scenario Mandy might think about talking to the doctor and theatre staff herself to take responsibility for the omission. She is likely to reflect on the circumstances that led her to forget and what she might have done differently and how to avoid the omission in the future. Her initial response was to get upset when confronted by the ward manager, but thereafter she might have regained her confidence from having thought things through and reflecting on how to do things differently.

Scenario: Whose accountability? (page 14)

In this scenario Mandy might reflect on what led her to identify the near miss. Sarah might reflect on the assessment of the patient, interprofessional communication, pharmacological knowledge and patient collaboration in care planning. In this scenario Mandy was responsible for completing the delegated task of preparing the patient for discharge and for reporting new information and any concerns. Sarah was accountable for acting on that information and for overseeing the care Mandy gave to the patient, including any drugs to take home. Mandy is likely to have learned that she has good assessment and observation skills that helped her to check information appropriately. Sarah might have learned that, no matter how experienced, professionals are fallible. She may also have learned that students can help to interrogate practice.

Documenting reflection

To help document some of the reflection that you might have undertaken in completing the activities in this chapter, you might want to consider:

- description of experience;
- evaluation;
- analysis;
- future action.

The following pro forma is offered to help you begin to document reflection.

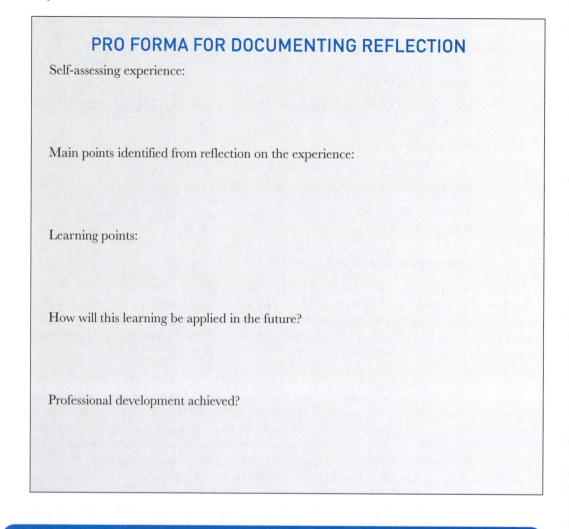

PRO FORMA FOR DOCUMENTING REFLECTION

Self-assessing experience:

Main points identified from reflection on the experience:

Learning points:

How will this learning be applied in the future?

Professional development achieved?

Further reading

Richardson, R (2008) *Clinical Skills for Student Nurses: Theory, practice and reflection.* Exeter: Reflect Press.

This book links the NMC Essential Skills Clusters with learning clinical skills and reflecting on those processes.

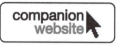

For further activities and other useful material, visit the companion website at **www.sagepub.co.uk/howatson-jones_reflective2e**

Chapter 2
Lifewide and lifelong learning and reflection

NMC Standards for Pre-registration Nursing Education

This chapter will address the following competencies:

Domain 1: Professional values

7. All nurses must be responsible and accountable for keeping their knowledge and skills up to date through continuing professional development. They must aim to improve their performance and enhance the safety and quality of care through evaluation, supervision and appraisal.

8. All nurses must practise independently, recognising the limits of their competence and knowledge. They must reflect on these limits and seek advice from, or refer to, other professionals where necessary.

NMC Essential Skills Clusters

This chapter will address the following ESCs:

Cluster: Organisational aspects of care

15. People can trust a newly registered graduate nurse to safely delegate to others and to respond appropriately when a task is delegated to them.

By the first progression point:

1. Accepts delegated activities within limitations of own role, knowledge and skill.

Cluster: Infection prevention and control

22. People can trust the newly registered graduate nurse to maintain effective standard infection control precautions and apply and adapt these to needs and limitations in all environments.

By the first progression point:

1. Demonstrates effective hand hygiene and the appropriate use of standard infection control precautions when caring for all people.

Chapter aims

By the end of this chapter you will be able to:

- define what is meant by lifewide and lifelong learning;
- identify some of the contexts in which learning takes place;
- identify features of learning in formal and less formal ways;
- consider types of knowledge and ways of knowing;
- understand how the person learns through reflection.

Example story

Jenny had finished her first placement in her second year of the nurse preparation programme and was back in the university studying her next module. The module was about acute care. During the module the tutor explained the need for vigilant assessment and the students were asked to investigate a variety of techniques and tools to enable this to be undertaken and which encompassed a number of body systems. The scenarios offered were of mainstream surgical, medical and emergency situations that allowed the class to apply some of these strategies and techniques.

Jenny's placement had been in Radiology, where she had observed a number of procedures such as an **aortic stent insertion** and **uterine embolisation**. These were relatively new procedures, offering alternatives to more invasive and major interventions, such as surgical aortic aneurysm repair and hysterectomy. Jenny reflected on ways in which some of the assessment principles might be relevant to this different environment and different groups of patients. She noted that, although the procedures were less invasive, nevertheless they still represented acute care in that the patient was sedated and vulnerable to sudden major haemorrhage. Jenny discussed these different scenarios with her group during the group work and identified how the assessment strategies might be applied.

When the group was asked to give feedback about their work to the rest of the class, Jenny offered these alternative scenarios to help illustrate problem solving and application in a different care setting that, nevertheless, dealt with acute episodes within care. The tutor invited Jenny to explain more about the procedures in order to help expand the knowledge of the whole class – and her own, as she was not as intimately familiar with the practice of the procedures as Jenny had been.

When reflecting upon this after class, Jenny realised that, no matter how knowledgeable a person may be, learning does not stop with a qualification. Equally, by explaining her learning about the procedures to others, Jenny was able also to perceive some gaps in her knowledge in terms of the assessment strategies and tools at her disposal.

Introduction

Learning can be defined as multi-dimensional in terms of where and how it takes place. Yet, learning is also a very individual process and what is carried forward may, perhaps, only truly be gauged by the person themselves. What is grasped may not always be what is taught. In the example story offered at the beginning of this chapter, what is grasped is the need to assert a knowledge base, even if this differs from the examples being taught. The quality of the response received may influence whether this learning is taken forward or inhibited. To take ownership of learning requires an understanding of where and how learning can take place.

This chapter will emphasise that learning does not only take place through formal courses or instruction, but extends into all areas of life, a theme that is taken forward in the subsequent chapter. This chapter begins by defining what is meant by lifewide and lifelong learning, and offers an example of each. The contexts in which nurses might learn are explored and considered in terms of their levels of formality and the learner's autonomy to design some aspects of their own learning. The chapter identifies different types of knowledge, how nurses come to know, and how this relates to reflection. It concludes by summarising the relationship between reflection and lifelong learning.

Throughout the chapter, you will be invited to complete a variety of activities and consider a number of case studies and scenarios to enable you to examine the different contexts of your learning and analyse progression of your learning.

What is lifewide learning?

Lifewide learning is learning that is not only limited to the classroom, but extends into many other areas of life (West et al., 2007). Lifewide learning includes informal discussion, interest activities and learning within the family (Field, 2006). For example, we often discuss our views with others and in the process might learn a different perspective on a problem from their response, or even some new knowledge that they have learned and that they share with us. Becoming involved in an activity, such as sport, may involve learning the rules of the game or new techniques. Family life involves a multitude of skills and tasks, with learning available to the family members according to family **culture** and tradition. Equally, incidental learning may occur during your formal preparation programme: for example, learning to type and word process, managing your time and developing professional attitudes. These may not be taught formally, but are aspects that you are likely to absorb as part of completing the programme. As a learner you are able to define the different aspects of your life that contribute to your learning. Consider the following case study of Paul's difficult encounter as an example of informal learning taking place within his social peer group.

Case study: Paul's difficult encounter

Paul was in the third year of his nurse preparation programme. He lived in a rented house with two friends who were also on the programme. Paul was working in accident and emergency. During his shift one day, he had looked after a 13-year-old girl who had been brought in after taking an overdose of paracetamol. After recording her observations he had tried to get hold of her mother. When her mother did arrive she started shouting at her daughter, saying she was sick of her constant attention seeking and that she was going to put her into care. The mother and daughter were shouting so much that Paul had to ask the mother to wait in the waiting room. She replied that she washed her hands of her daughter and left. Paul was shocked and upset by this episode and came home troubled by it.

In the evening he broached the subject with his housemates, talking about the case but leaving out the names. He told them how he could not understand the mother's reaction. Why would she want to put her child into care? He wondered whether the reason the daughter had taken the overdose was because she felt unloved by her mother. He had also been disquieted by the reaction of some of the qualified staff who appeared not to take the girl seriously.

During their discussion it became clear that Paul's housemates had some alternative views that stemmed from their different experiences. They suggested that there might be a number of reasons for the mother's reaction. Stress and exhaustion were obvious ones, if she felt she simply could not cope any longer. Paul's friend Rob explained how he had had a friend at school who would self-harm because of the pressure his stepfather put on him. At first he could not understand it, until his friend explained that it was a bit like opening a release valve. The other housemate, Alex, who was undertaking the Mental Health nurse preparation programme, suggested that the mother and daughter might have been projecting behaviour on to each other because of the pain they were both experiencing. What he was trying to explain was that people can be manipulative for a number of reasons, not least because of the pain they feel and poor self-esteem. Paul was thoughtful after this discussion and considered that perhaps his initial view was too simplistic. Projection was not something he knew much about and he thought it might be useful to explore further. He decided to read up on it to develop his understanding.

Having read this case study you might have also questioned the daughter's and mother's actions. In addition, you might have perceived how the informal discussion within his house group developed Paul's thinking. By completing Activity 2.1 you will be able to review your own lifewide learning.

Activity 2.1   *Critical thinking*

Develop a map of your learning that extends beyond classroom-based learning. You might want to consider situations involving:

- social learning;
- self-designed learning;
- leisure pursuit learning;
- family learning.

There is some guidance about this activity at the end of the chapter.

The map of your learning is likely to have helped to illustrate how extensive your learning might actually be when considered outside the confines of the classroom and within the extent of your life. Examining your learning in this way helps to analyse its progression. We now proceed to consider the relationship to lifelong learning.

What is lifelong learning?

Lifelong learning refers to a process of learning that continues across our lives (Jarvis, 2010). Lifelong learning is a professional reality for nurses because healthcare and the technologies that support it are constantly evolving. It is for this reason that lifelong learning in healthcare often takes the form of practice development (Mason-Whitehead and Mason, 2008). The NMC (2008), through the professional code for nurses and midwives, advocates that nurses continue to learn not only to maintain the currency of their knowledge, but to have an enquiring attitude to their practice and performance. This is also part of the standard of professional values as presented at the start of this chapter, and requires you to be open to new experiences while recognising limitations to your knowledge and doing something about them. Thus, lifelong learning comes with an individual responsibility to pursue learning as well as being part of your preparation programme. Lifelong learning differs from lifelong education in that learning is about developing your understanding across the spectrum of your life, while education might be assumed to refer to the ways these ideas might be taught (Jarvis, 2010).

Healthcare draws particularly on knowledge relating to the body and ways of doing things that also have an emotional and social dimension when working with people (Twigg, 2006). Lifelong aspects of learning also relate to who you are within your relationships with people, which is linked to the culture you have grown up in, your history, hopes and ideas, as well as your goals. For example, how does your experience of learning in its widest sense influence your approaches to ongoing learning? This might relate to the way emotional aspects of learning, with regard to the feelings produced by past learning experiences, are taken forward, influencing your engagement with further learning and remembering what you have learned. Lifelong learning in a lifewide sense invites an approach to learning that includes others in how they have influenced you (West et al., 2007). Learning involves social elements through our interactions, emotional aspects perceived by how we feel about things, and cognitive parts representing our thinking (Illeris, 2004). These all have an influence on our sense of self and our learning.

Lifelong learning also encompasses a number of dimensions that interconnect according to your intentions and opportunities, as illustrated in Figure 2.1.

Formal learning is usually directed towards a learning outcome. For example, your nurse preparation programme is based on a curriculum covering what you need to know to work as a registered nurse. This curriculum has been verified by the regulatory body. The outcome is being able to function as a registered nurse at the end of the programme. Informal learning relates to the discussions you may have with your peers and patients, which also help to develop your thinking and knowledge. Relationship-centred learning is about how you learn to manage attitudes and feelings within your encounters with others. Experiential learning relates to what

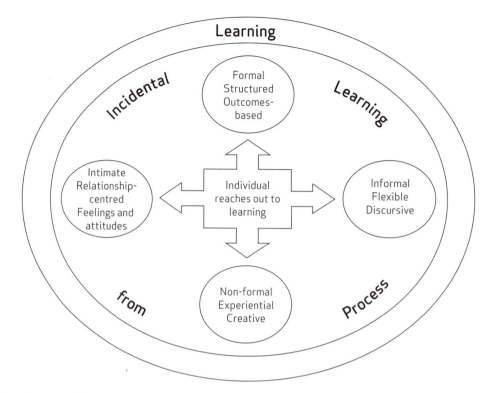

Figure 2.1: Some dimensions of learning

you learn from dealing with different situations. Incidental learning occurs alongside all of these activities and is influenced by the quality of these experiences.

You, as an individual, are at the centre of your learning, as it is up to you whether you actually engage with it and discern what you have learned. How you integrate different ways of learning is another form of learning itself and a major part of lifelong learning. To do this involves reflecting on your learning and possible connections between different forms of learning, and on your development as part of the analysis process. Consider the case study involving Shuki's integration of her learning in order to identify how such reflectively integrated learning might contribute to further learning.

Case study: Shuki's integration of her learning

Shuki came from an Indian family where she was the middle child of five siblings. As both her parents worked, she had often helped with her siblings and consequently learned the skills of looking after herself at the same time. To her, a nursing qualification was important to enable her to support herself and contribute to the family.

Shuki was in the first year of her nurse preparation programme and was learning about the human body, the fundamentals of practice and her developing professional identity. She enjoyed the practical aspects of the course as she could connect some of what she was learning to her previous knowledge of caring for her siblings in terms of hygiene and bathing, feeding and elimination. Shuki did find some of the theoretical elements hard to

continued . . .

grasp, especially the clinical science sessions, which seemed so full of jargon that she did not really understand. Shuki reflected on what she could do.

When she thought about it, Shuki equated the problem to learning a different language. At home she spoke an Indian dialect and English, and remembered how she had found it easier to learn English from her friends. Maybe she could draw on her bilingual experiences to help her to learn this scientific language. Shuki decided this would be easier if she could share this with others and so asked some of her class if they wanted to form a revision group. They agreed to meet, on an informal basis, before class on Thursday for two hours to go over what they had learned in the previous session and to fill in the gaps. Shuki was surprised and pleased at her success in arranging this group. When she reflected on this she also recognised that some of her experiences of managing herself were also instrumental in this organisation and design of her learning and of her developing assertiveness. By drawing together different threads of her learning she was also able to contribute to her further learning.

Having read this case study you might have started to reflect on your own lifelong learning and how different aspects might connect to make something new. Try to analyse what this might mean for you. Undertaking Activity 2.2 offers you an opportunity to think about your lifelong learning and reach some conclusions.

Activity 2.2   *Reflection*

Think about your learning since you started your nurse preparation programme. If you are in your first year of the course you might want to consider the following questions.

- How has my view of nursing changed and why?
- What skills have I learned?
- How has my identity changed?

If you are further on in your nurse preparation programme you might want to think about the following.

- What areas of my knowledge have changed and why?
- What areas of my knowledge do I need to develop further and why?

If you are an experienced practitioner you might want to think about the following.

- What changes have happened in healthcare since I started in my practitioner role?
- What knowledge change has this required from me?
- How did I develop this knowledge?
- What further goals do I have for my learning?

There is some guidance about this activity at the end of the chapter.

When completing this activity you might have considered different contexts and ways in which you increased your knowledge during your nurse preparation programme and over time. We now proceed to look at some contexts in which learning takes place.

Contexts in which learning takes place

The theoretical learning that you undertake in university helps to inform your practice, just as your practice can also help to inform theory when something new is identified in the way that perhaps a patient responds to the interventions you are involved in. Your placements are another context for learning from the experiences you have there. Patients are all different, and so are the contexts in which they are nursed. Each of these experiences offers an opportunity for learning.

Learning, whether undertaken in university or in practice, can also be shared with others. Learning as a group is a valuable way of turning ideas into articulated thinking. Explaining something to someone else shows us what we really understand about an issue and, at the same time, the feedback from others opens up the possibilities of thinking further to develop understanding. The virtual world may provide another avenue for expanding our ideas and learning when others are not immediately available to converse with or to share ideas with.

The virtual world can be both a public and private space for learning. For example, virtual learning environment (VLE) discussion boards may be viewed by many course participants and are public. Contributions may, correspondingly, be less spontaneous and more thought through before being placed in such a public domain because of possible concerns with and anticipation of others' reactions (Kozlowski, 2002). In this context it is sometimes harder to acknowledge unfinished thinking. Nevertheless, electronic resources also provide opportunities for learning that is individually focused. For example, you can look up the action of a particular drug or disease process, or identify the latest research underpinning a particular nursing intervention. This learning can be accessed and completed in private and at your own pace.

There may also be times when you are too shy to ask, and it may be tempting to rely solely on such sources for information that do not expose you to the scrutiny of others. However, it is important to remember that not all electronic sources or sites are credible and some information may also be biased. You are referred to *Information Skills for Nursing Students* (Hutchfield, 2010) in this series for greater guidance on using electronic resources and virtual environments for learning. It is important to make sure that such learning is related to some framework for learning to help you to stay focused. You will also need to have access to reliable guidance to help evaluate what you have found in order to avoid mistakes. An example might be looking something up and then discussing this further with your mentor or course tutor. This not only helps to avoid mistakes, but also may help to share learning that is beneficial with others.

When trying anything for the first time there is an element of learning from the mistakes you might make. Mistakes can be a valuable way of learning when you reflect on what went wrong, analyse the processes that led to the mistake and consider what you can do to avoid making the same mistake another time. Taking responsibility for what has gone wrong enables new ideas to develop (Rogers and Freiberg, 1994). Mistakes, although unpleasant in their possible consequences and challenges to self-esteem, also provide emotional learning about how to deal with anxiety and disappointment, and move on more positively. Support for such learning may come from family members or close peers, as well as through the encouragement of colleagues. Nevertheless, this requires time to really reflect on what has been learned. To help you understand some of these points relating to learning from mistakes, consider the following scenario.

Scenario: Jon's mistake

Jon was working in a nursing home and was in his first year of the nurse preparation programme. He had been working in the home for three weeks and was getting to know the residents better. He liked working with them as they often had interesting stories to tell about their earlier lives. Jon was using this opportunity to also put into practice some of the skills he had learned in his clinical skills sessions, such as handwashing and bed bathing. Although the majority of the residents only needed some help with personal care, there was one man – Harry – who had had a stroke and needed considerably more help. He had also had some loose stools a few days earlier and was feeling rather weak.

Jon was looking after Harry today and offered to help give him a bed bath as the matron wanted to avoid Harry using the main bath until his bowel motions were back to normal. Jon had undertaken a few bed baths with his mentor, but as the opportunity did not arise very often Jon was keen to undertake this. He gathered all the necessary equipment together and shut the door to Harry's room to ensure privacy. While he was helping Harry to remove his pyjamas, Jon conversed with him about Harry's time in the army. Harry started to tell Jon a funny story about an escapade he and his friends had arranged when they were on their training course.

At the end of the bed bath Jon asked his mentor to help him to dress Harry again and help him to sit out in his chair for a little while. It was only when he was putting everything away that Jon realised that he had forgotten to change the water, although he had changed the wash cloth between the general and intimate areas. Jon told his mentor and how terrible he felt about the mistake. Jon's mentor asked him to reflect on the process that he had gone through when undertaking the bed bath and the possible consequences for Harry of not changing the water.

Jon reflected on the order in which he had helped Harry to wash particular areas of his body. He also thought about when he changed the wash cloth and his reasoning for this. Jon also considered the purpose and requirements for changing the water. Jon told his mentor that he had helped Harry to wash his front first including his genitalia, as this included Harry in his own care. Jon realised that he had then proceeded to wash Harry's back, bottom and legs. He had used a different cloth for Harry's bottom, but the same water was used for his legs. Jon's mentor identified that it was better practice to wash intimate areas separately. This was especially important because of Harry's recent history of loose stools. She asked Jon to consider why he forgot to change the water. Jon realised that he had been distracted by the conversation. This led Jon to consider how in future he would manage the therapeutic relationship at the same time as completing care correctly.

Questions
- What are the significant aspects of this scenario and why?
- Why is it important for Jon to reflect on the actions that he undertook during the bed bath?

If you are an experienced practitioner think about what you want to consider as the mentor.

There are outline answers to these questions at the end of the chapter.

This scenario may have identified some of the difficulties involved for the novice practitioner in trying to maintain a therapeutic relationship while completing actions accurately. Both of these are contexts of learning and we need to be able to reconcile the formal and the less formal. We now proceed to consider some features of formal and less formal ways of learning.

Features of learning in formal and less formal ways

Features of formal learning involve codifying information into our thinking (Eraut, 2001). What this means is that the information is often offered already in the form of categories and theories, which we embed in our thinking according to particular required outcomes. This may make concepts easier to grasp, but at the same time might also inhibit the development of different interpretations. Reflecting on formal learning can help to negate such effects by opening up alternative views. Consider some features in your formal learning by completing Activity 2.3.

Activity 2.3   *Critical thinking*

Think about a recent class you attended as part of your nurse preparation programme. What features of learning can you identify by considering the following questions.

- How did the lesson start?
- What were you asked to do during the lesson?
- How did the lesson finish?
- What did you learn?
- Did you do anything further to aid your learning after the lesson and, if so, what did you do?

If you are an experienced practitioner consider a recent CPD session.

There is an outline answer to this activity at the end of the chapter.

Formal learning may help to provide some knowledge for practice and begin the process of professional learning. Sharing experiences is an important feature of professional learning in less formal ways. Different interpretations based on subjective experiences may be offered and explored, allowing debate and reconsideration of the conclusions that might be reached. The features of this learning are its evolving and discursive nature, which means that it is flexible and responsive, but therefore also harder to quantify and evidence. Personal learning can also help to support professional practice and is another feature of less formal ways of learning through reworking personal knowledge within the professional setting. An example might be having the ability to speak another language and using this to translate in the professional setting. Integrating personal and professional learning supports a holistic approach to health and social care. Consider some features of your less formal learning by completing Activity 2.4.

Activity 2.4   *Critical thinking*

Think about a recent discussion you had in practice. What features of learning can you identify by examining the following.

*   What prompted the discussion?
*   What were the key arguments made?
*   What was the outcome of the discussion?
*   What did you learn?
*   Did you do anything further to aid your learning?

There is an outline answer to this activity at the end of the chapter.

Within these two activities you will have had an opportunity to compare and contrast different forms of learning. We now proceed to look at types of knowledge and ways of knowing that are relevant to the healthcare practitioner.

Types of knowledge and ways of knowing

Theories and protocols – what Eraut (2001) calls propositional knowledge – are important for identifying what knowledge is expected of the professional learner. Examples include theories of communication and psychological processing, how the human body works, disease effects, infection control and much more. Protocols relate to identification of what is required within a particular procedure. Examples of these might be assessment procedures, what to do when someone suffers a stroke or cardiac arrest, or how to prepare somebody for an operation and so on. This constitutes professional knowledge, with professional ways of knowing relating to the meaning that a professional derives from situations through experience and applying theory to practice.

Practical knowledge relates to knowing how to do things and developing the skills required to carry them out. This knowledge is part of the *professional craft* (Titchen et al., 2004, p108). Personal knowledge comes from the **lifeworld** of the individual (Jarvis, 2006). That means that it comes from their background, culture, who they interact with and the activities in which they are involved. It relates also to how individuals see themselves and others. Personal knowledge develops from reflecting on events and making sense of situations. Layers of experience may filter into the unconscious until re-emerging as intuitive knowing. The following short case study is offered as an example of how the different types of knowledge and knowing may all interlink in your practice of healthcare.

Case study: Suzy's day

*Suzy was in her last year of the nurse preparation programme. She was working in an **oncology** setting, which she enjoyed. There were clear guidelines for when patients were due to have particular treatments, and Suzy had spent today discussing some of these with her mentor, Ben, in order to gain a better*

continued . . .

understanding. Ben had first explored Suzy's knowledge of the relevant clinical science relating to various types of cancers, in particular the cell development cycle and how this was important to determine treatment phases.

The discussion between Suzy and Ben then moved forward to her assessment, which was due soon. Suzy identified that many of the patients required regular blood tests and, although Suzy had been trained in **venepuncture** *in her previous role as a health care assistant (HCA), she understood that she was not allowed to undertake this in her current role as a student because of differences in responsibility and accountability. Ben highlighted, however, that Suzy was always ready with the required equipment when other nurses needed to take a sample, which they valued. She had also been quick to identify* **phlebitis** *in a patient, which was undoubtedly due to her previous experience.*

Ben asked Suzy to reflect on why she enjoyed working in this particular setting and what she thought she had learned. When thinking about this, Suzy identified that dignity, respect and compassion were important values for her. Supporting people with cancer was fulfilling for her because of the opportunity to really listen and attend to someone else's situation, as she was not able to be involved in some of the treatments. From this she had learned what therapeutic relationship and communication might actually mean in practice and not just as an abstract idea.

Through reading the case study you may have noted how professional, practical and personal knowledge may be integrated in a typical day. The role of reflection in achieving this is paramount. We finish this chapter by highlighting how learning is related to reflection.

Learning and reflection

Processes of learning can carry mixed emotions that can get in the way of learning experiences, because of the anxiety that might be aroused. Learning reams of facts also does not embed understanding or application of learning. In order to transform learning into something that you can apply in different situations with different people and at different times, reflection on learning is required in order to examine what has actually been learned. It is through reflection that connections can be made between:

- lifewide and lifelong learning;
- different types of learning;
- different types of knowledge and knowing;
- how to deal with emotions;
- what values and beliefs are developing;
- what alternatives are available;
- what are the likely outcomes;
- what nursing is.

> ## Chapter summary
>
> This chapter has started to examine some of the issues listed above and offered a variety of opportunities to make some of these connections through the case studies, activities and scenarios provided. Through these it has been possible for you to apply some of the ideas around lifewide and lifelong learning in different settings and at different stages of the nurse preparation programme. This is a crucial part of continuing lifelong learning as set out in the NMC standards at the start of the chapter, as healthcare continues to evolve and change. How to explore lifewide learning in greater depth is the subject of the next chapter.

Activities and scenarios: Brief outline answers

Activity 2.1: Critical thinking (page 22)

Your answer might have included:

- how to communicate in different groupings;
- developing friendships;
- using the internet to find information, writing up notes, reading;
- learning to drive, swim, play a sport;
- learning to cook, manage finance, become a parent.

You might have found it helpful to develop a visual map of all your learning first and then to group various categories together.

Activity 2.2: Reflection (page 25)

If you are a novice practitioner in your first year, your answer might have considered that:

- nursing is hard work and emotionally challenging;
- skills learned in the first year include recording nursing observations such as temperature, pulse, respiration and blood pressure and oxygen saturations, and undertaking urinalysis, bed bathing, simple wound care, administering injections, checking medications with the mentor, caring for urinary catheters;
- identity changes might include becoming more assertive and confident.

If you are further on in your nurse preparation programme, you might have thought about:

- having more knowledge about how clinical science applies in practice;
- a need to develop wider knowledge of pharmacology and pathophysiology in order to understand treatment options.

If you are an experienced practitioner, you might have thought about:

- increasing use of technology in nursing observations and interventions;
- the move to an all-graduate profession for nursing;
- returning to further formal academic study;
- investigating new opportunities and knowledge requirements in nursing.

Activity 2.3: Critical thinking (page 28)

Your answer might have identified that the lesson started with the learning objectives of what was expected for you to learn. You might have been asked to discuss some of the concepts in smaller groups and apply these to practice scenarios. The lesson might have finished by summarising the main points. You might have identified that you remembered some of the key points and might have undertaken some further reading of your notes.

As an experienced practitioner thinking about a CPD session, you might have considered how the lesson started by enquiring about your present knowledge of the topic. During the session you are likely to have discussed application to your practice, in small groups. The session could have finished with a summary of the key points and guidance on directed study. You might have tried to fit in the directed study around your workload and expanded your learning through further discussion with work colleagues.

Activity 2.4: Critical thinking (page 29)

Your answer might have identified that a patient problem stimulated the discussion. Key points of this discussion are likely to have included some background information about the problem, who needed to be involved and possible solutions. The outcome is likely to have been an agreement on the solution to be implemented. You might have identified learning about decision making, team working and problem solving. You might have reflected on this further afterwards. Have you noticed that it seems more natural to reflect on situations that are based on relationships?

Scenario: Jon's mistake (page 27)

The significant aspects of this scenario are the problem with maintaining focus while multi-tasking and the risk of cross-contamination because of the lapse in concentration. Good hygiene is vital when diarrhoea is suspected, to avoid its rapid spread and introducing organisms to other areas of the body. Jon needed to reflect on how he managed communication while undertaking care and the order in which he had completed the bed bath and why he had chosen this sequence. Both Jon and his mentor needed to review his knowledge base and redress any deficits. It would also be important for Jon's mentor to help him to repair his self-esteem. This might be achieved by his mentor helping Jon to identify the positive aspects of his communication.

As an experienced practitioner thinking as a mentor you might consider:

* how to maintain a supportive learning relationship while correcting practice;
* how to construct feedback to support safe and effective practice;
* how to act on the learning results.

Further reading

Hutchfield, K (2010) *Information Skills for Nursing Students.* Exeter: Learning Matters.

This is an easy guide to using electronic media.

Mason-Whitehead, E and **Mason, T** (2008) *Study Skills for Nurses,* 2nd edition. Los Angeles, CA: Sage.

This book has a useful section on lifelong learning that includes the formal and less formal. It also relates lifelong learning to continuing career development when the nurse preparation programme has been completed.

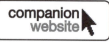

For further activities and other useful material, visit the companion website at **www.sagepub.co.uk/howatson-jones_reflective2e**

Chapter 3
Autobiographical reflection and learning

NMC Standards for Pre-registration Nursing Education

This chapter will address the following competencies:

Domain 1: Professional values

8. All nurses must practise independently, recognising the limits of their competence and knowledge. They must reflect on these limits and seek advice from, or refer to, other professionals where necessary.

Domain 4: Leadership, management and team working

4. All nurses must be self-aware and recognise how their own values, principles and assumptions may affect their practice. They must maintain their own personal and professional development, learning from experience, through supervision, feedback, reflection and evaluation.

NMC Essential Skills Clusters

This chapter will address the following ESCs:

Cluster: Care, compassion and communication

5. People can trust the newly registered, graduate nurse to engage with them in a warm, sensitive and compassionate way.

By the first progression point:

5. Evaluates ways in which own interactions affect relationships to ensure that they do not impact inappropriately on others.

Cluster: Organisational aspects of care

10. People can trust the newly registered graduate nurse to deliver nursing interventions and evaluate their effectiveness against the agreed assessment and care plan.

By the second progression point:

4. Actively seeks to extend knowledge and skills using a variety of methods in order to enhance care delivery.

11. People can trust the newly registered graduate nurse to safeguard children and adults from vulnerable situations and support and protect them from harm.

By the first progression point:

3. Uses support systems to recognise, manage and deal with own emotions.

Chapter aims

After reading this chapter you will be able to:

- consider how reflection integrates the personal with the professional, drawing on experiences from all areas of life;
- complete a life story construction exercise;
- creatively explore your experiences by reflecting upon your autobiography;
- integrate autobiographical reflection and learning with a sense of a developing identity;
- reflect on aspects of your life that may also be revealing of societal issues.

Example story

Lizzie came from a large family. She had three older siblings and two younger. Her parents both worked. Her older brothers had left home and her sister, who was in her late teens, was intent on pursuing her own social life. One night, when she was 16, Lizzie offered to stay with her younger siblings so that her parents could go out for a meal to celebrate her mother's birthday. Her younger brother and sister were 12 and 8 respectively at the time, so it was not too much of a hardship to keep an eye on them.

While playing an electronic game with her brother, Lizzie noticed that her sister Amy was looking very tired and becoming distressed with the flashing lights and loud noises from the game. She suggested that Amy might be better going to bed. When she went to say goodnight to Amy she noticed that she looked very pale. Amy pulled up her pyjama top and showed Lizzie a collection of spots on her abdomen. Lizzie remembered an advertisement for the warning signs of meningitis that she had seen on the television. She got a glass and rolled it over the spots. They did not fade. She also noted that, earlier, Amy had been avoiding the lights and noises of the game. Lizzie took action, calling her parents and an ambulance. It was later confirmed that Amy did indeed have meningitis and that Lizzie's vigilance had ensured she received treatment early. Her parents were full of praise. Lizzie felt emotionally confused, happy that her sister was recovering, but also guilty that she had not noticed earlier.

A few years later, no one was surprised that Lizzie chose to become a children's nurse. When she was writing her statement for consideration for entry to the programme, Lizzie reflected on this episode in order to identify some of her attributes. She concluded that she had the observational and decision-making skills required of a nurse, but also considered that this episode had taught her that there were emotional consequences to caring work.

As a student practitioner, Lizzie has reflected further on how the emotional residue from caring work may be different when dealing with situations personally or professionally. She has used her autobiographical experience to develop discussion with her peers about the observation of symptoms and disease as well as the emotional consequences of critical incidents. Through sharing this story she has come to a better understanding of herself as a capable and caring person who copes well in critical situations, but who also requires emotional support to work through her thinking.

Introduction

This chapter has started with an example story to help illustrate how autobiographical experience can assist student nurse practitioners to make sense of their capabilities and progress. You will have entered into your professional preparation programme with a variety of experiences. These will influence your perception and experience of yourself, of others and of practice. Developing reflective insight is an important starting point for any professional entering into a caring profession, and particularly for nursing. Such insight explains why we react and think in certain ways, what resources in the form of family and friends and personal knowledge are available to us, and what the possibilities might be for development and change.

This chapter introduces the idea of autobiographical reflection as a way to advance nursing knowledge in different ways. It will first define what autobiographical reflection is before proceeding to consider how to integrate personal and professional experience and the importance of doing so. You will be invited to construct your own autobiography with guidance on the key points for inclusion in the construction. This is followed by further guidance on how to examine and reflect on your autobiography. The chapter ends by looking at how societal issues may be given meaning through subjective experience.

What is autobiographical reflection?

As people progress through life they begin to develop a life history. This history, just like any other, charts the timeline of events and the changes that have come about. It also includes motives for particular actions, how situations have been shaped, how the individual has been shaped by events and their aspirations for the future. From the experiences that individuals have in their lives, personal knowledge develops. Experiences may be very diverse, as they result from the ways in which we come into contact with the world and make sense of it through interacting with it (Boud and Miller, 1996). For example, going to school exposes an individual to many different people and types of learning. Others' reactions to efforts made at interacting and understanding provide feedback that is internalised as knowledge of personal ability. Read the following scenario of David's biographical account of school to identify what learning he might have taken forward from this experience.

Scenario: David's biographical account of school

David went to a mixed comprehensive school. He was really good at science, but had limited social skills and found it difficult to interact with others because he had Asperger's syndrome. People with Asperger's can have difficulty with reading social cues and processing language. David's class mates often made fun of him. He excelled in drama and science and put his science knowledge to good use doing the lighting for school productions. He liked working behind the scenes rather than presenting in public. David achieved mixed exam results and had to retake some of them. As a consequence his self-esteem suffered. David's teacher was aware of his needs and was very supportive. She gave David space to talk about his experience and then asked him to help another boy, Jonathan, to revise for his exam resits. Jonathan had dyslexia and she thought David's methodical approach might help him and raise David's own self-esteem and confidence. Both David and Jonathan passed their resits and considered what to do next. They discussed caring work as they had enjoyed working together. They both applied to study nursing.

Question

*   What learning is David taking forward from school?

See the notes on Activity 3.1 at the end of the chapter for an answer to this question.

The scenario above identifies that school experiences can be both positive and challenging. Horsdal (2012, p25) suggests that the way we use our senses and communicate affects the development of our 'social brain'. Sharing our experiences with an empathic listener, such as David did with his teacher, means that we are able to retrace our paths in a supported way and consequently learn from our experiences. In such a way experiences can be transformed through autobiographical reflection. An autobiography turns these experiences into an account of what has been lived through and the meaning that has been attached to this as part of a personal history. An autobiographical reflection is different in its focus from a more traditional reflection. Autobiography reviews individual experiences within the life history and reflection scrutinises links between them to explore how the past might be influencing the present. In doing so it finds creative ways to address situations and problems by drawing on personal knowledge that has come from a personal history. In this way autobiographical reflection helps to make sense of past experiences within an individual life history and what might be being taken forward, raising the possibility of change.

We do not always pay attention to the experiences that we come into contact with and therefore may not recognise their value in terms of what has been learned and what can be translated into different circumstances and situations. Equally, there may be times when it feels like we have reached an impasse by perhaps becoming too overwhelmed by the situation to be able to move forward. For example, learning anatomy and physiology can be difficult for some people and yet these are integral parts of nursing knowledge. If you have artistic attributes these will potentially play a part in how you perceive things and possibly respond to them. You may be more drawn to the art of nursing than perhaps the science. Understanding this is a first step to dealing with potential difficulties that might arise in learning the language and structure of scientific theories.

Autobiographical reflection is a way of making sense of what is happening, set within the context of a person's life, by focusing attention on that person's life history to identify how the person can renegotiate a position and deal with the challenge (Horsdal, 2007). This renegotiation is called 'agency', by which individuals are able to take control of their lives. Individuals use their life resources to construct strategies for developing and dealing with change (West et al., 2007). Therefore, in the example of the artistic student nurse, it might be that developing revision notes that use colour and drawing is one way to surmount the obstacle to understanding scientific concepts. As stated by Boud et al. (1985, p19), reflection in the first instance requires:

- returning to experience;
- attending to feelings;
- re-evaluating experience.

Activity 3.1   *Reflection*

Look back at the scenario of David's biographical account of school and consider the following.

- What meaning do you think he has attached to his experiences?
- What creative ways might he find to help his learning?

There is an outline answer to this activity at the end of the chapter.

Autobiographical reflection explores personal learning in how the past is combined with perceptions of sensations within the present (Jarvis, 2007). Such reflection involves thinking about how, in the first instance, to construct the autobiographical account in terms of what to include, and what seems relevant in the present moment and why. For example, it can be helpful to gather autobiographical experiences of learning – what Dominice (2000) calls *writing an educational biography* – in order to develop an understanding of personal learning processes by reflecting on diverse learning experience through the life history. Such autobiographical reflection looks at learning in its widest sense of formal and informal experience.

Apply consideration of autobiographical experience to your own life by completing Activity 3.2.

Activity 3.2   *Critical thinking*

Spend a little time thinking of a particular story from your life history and write it down.

- What made you think of that story?
- What feelings does the story bring back for you and why?
- Whose voices appear in the story and what are the relationships?
- What has changed between then and now?
- Can you think of ways in which writing your autobiography might help develop your learning?

There is some guidance on this activity at the end of the chapter.

Autobiographical reflection also requires acknowledging how we feel about the past, and this may be costly in terms of the emotional aspects that might appear. Being able to deal with your own emotions is one of the essential skills of being a nurse. Being able to acknowledge feelings and recognise what stimulates them and why is also a way of recognising our own humanity, an important aspect when entering a caring profession. Remaining detached can be another way of suppressing feelings from past situations that are still active within the present. Cultural values are another rich seam that can also be explored through autobiographical reflection.

Having explored what autobiographical reflection is, we now move on to consider how personal and professional experience might be integrated.

Integrating personal and professional experience

Personal experience is a rich resource that may not always be seen as relevant to professional life, or professional experience. Nevertheless, the skills and knowledge developed within personal experience are the foundation from which individuals develop their professional identity and skills. For example, some of the roles that people inhabit within their lives, such as being a parent, a member of a committee or community group, a community group leader, an activity teacher and so on, bring valuable experiences that can integrate with professional experience, to advance knowledge and practice in different ways, thereby enhancing knowledge and skills. Completing Activity 3.3 will help you to identify what different roles and experiences you can bring to that of being a student practitioner.

Activity 3.3   *Reflection*

The examples offered are not exhaustive and there are many others that bring equally valuable experience. Take some time at this point to consider what roles you occupy in your personal life and the different activities you are involved in. Make a list of these. Now consider how these might integrate with your student practitioner or professional life. Spend a little time reflecting on the following questions.

- What knowledge is used in fulfilling the role?
- Are any particular skills involved and, if so, what are they?
- How might these skills be translated into different situations?
- Where are there connections with the professional/student practitioner role?

There is an outline answer to this activity at the end of the chapter.

Having completed Activity 3.3, you now have a clearer idea of where to direct your reflection. Integrating personal and professional experience involves reflecting upon what each contributes and how they may relate to each other. It is within the integration that knowledge can be synthesised in more creative ways. For example, some of the knowledge developed through the parenting role is likely to include lifespan development, disease management, communication and negotiation, leadership, organisation, nutrition, first aid and learning. Integration involves connecting this with what is learned through the professional/student practitioner role and through reflecting imaginatively, identifying possibilities and ways of doing things.

Imagining is part of a process of putting oneself into as yet unknown situations, and considering actions and possible consequences. This might mean, when first entering into the nurse preparation programme, working from a position of personal experience and imagining how to respond within some of the situations discussed in class but not as yet experienced. 'Imaging' is a way of thinking about and questioning possibilities as part of development (Parse, 1998). Reflective imagining goes further by integrating the personal with the professional, identifying the required ideal response and what is the likely response through self-knowledge and moving to consider how to develop. This is given definition through reading Marc's biographical account.

Case study: Marc's biographical account

Marc is French by birth, but has been brought up in Britain since he was seven years old because his mother's second marriage was to a British man. He is single and volunteers for a charity helpline in his spare time.

Marc is at the end of his nurse preparation programme. As he prepares for registration he is thinking about a recent placement where he found he was able to integrate his personal and professional knowledge in a meaningful way. He was working with the district nurses and visited a young man who had been in a road traffic accident in which he lost his girlfriend, his leg and subsequently his job. Following surgery and coming home, the wound had broken down and was now taking a long time to heal. By coincidence the patient was also French, although he spoke reasonable English. On the district nursing visits to change the dressing Marc had noticed that the patient was becoming increasingly withdrawn.

Marc tried to imagine what it must be like to lose so much so suddenly. He thought that anxiety and depression were most likely to follow, but was uncertain how to approach this. He knew he had good communication skills from his charity helpline activity, but he was not a trained counsellor. He also knew that he could communicate in the patient's native language, which helped. He started by checking whether his understanding of how the patient was feeling was correct. He did not, however, have enough mental health knowledge to proceed further and suggested to his mentor that a referral might be helpful.

*Marc reflected on how often mental health and general nursing issues overlapped. He considered that it would be good development, both professionally and personally, to undertake a counselling course. This experience had helped him to recognise that by integrating his personal and professional knowledge he had been able to reach the patient in a more personal way. With **reflexivity**, the experience had also shown him where he could develop further.*

Marc's biographical account has illustrated how reflective imagining begins when we are uncertain of what to do. Uncertainties with unknown situations disturb the mind. Jarvis (2007, p11) calls this *disharmony*. This prompts the imagining referred to above. Connecting with others, reflecting and imagining are all part of thinking. Integrated thinking means acknowledging that all experience can be useful to inform activity and equally different activities help to inform integrated thinking. But thinking, as identified in Marc's account, can also create uncertainty and anxiety where gaps in knowledge are perceived. Reflection and imagining perceive such gaps, as well as becoming stimulated by uncertainty and anxiety. What people bring to experiences can be drawn together through processes of reflecting and imagining with others, expanding solutions. These processes are illustrated in Figure 3.1 to represent how learning that integrates personal experience with professional experience might occur.

Integration only becomes possible when the processes of disequilibrium and seeking further information have occurred, including consulting others. The reflective practitioner incorporates imagination to support new directions that take account of feedback. When all are completed, integrative thinking draws the parts together.

Integrative thinking uses meanings. The first consideration is how we give meaning to a situation and communicate this to others. If our meaning is rejected by others, we may conform to their meaning as observed from their behaviour. Marc, in his account, checks with the patient his interpretation of how the patient is feeling. When meaning is discussed, others' views may be taken into consideration and used to help translate concepts. Marc is able to identify that the patient's feelings potentially translate into a mental health issue that requires addressing. Nevertheless, where others' interpretations become the accepted meaning, this too may become fixed and conform to behavioural norms, for example by viewing mental health and general nursing as something entirely separate.

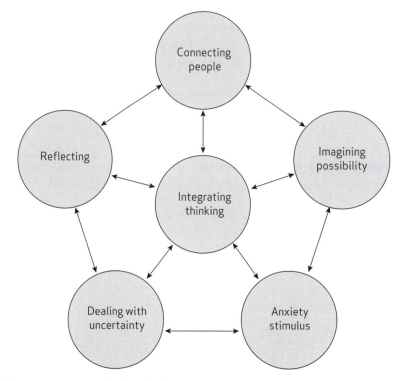

Figure 3.1: Integration of personal and professional experience
Source: Howatson-Jones (2010).

How anxiety is managed determines whether reflective imagination is restrained by conforming behaviours or enabled by ideas continuing to develop and reach out to the unknown, while considering reflexively how the self is changing. Anxiety is the stimulant to thinking of alternatives and experimenting with change, but needs to be accompanied by self-awareness of overcoming obstacles to support positive progress. For example, Marc's confidence has increased because his mentor has taken his concern seriously. These points are illustrated in a schema in Figure 3.2. The influence of anxiety is shown at the crossing points marked with an X and the arrows represent potential direction.

Review your own meaning making and development of ideas by completing Activity 3.4.

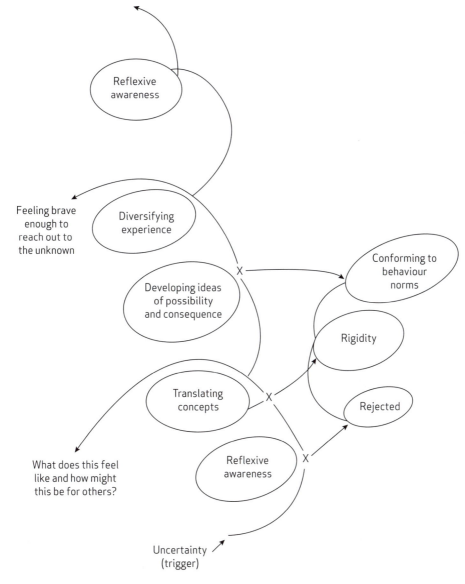

Figure 3.2: Schema of reflective imagination
Source: Howatson-Jones (2010).

There is an outline answer to this activity at the end of the chapter.

Activity 3.4	*Critical thinking*

- Looking back on your own life, identify a situation where you were anxious and uncertain of how to proceed, or where you were moving into a new beginning. You might consider coming on to your nurse preparation programme, or moving into your first qualified practitioner role when completing the programme.
- Reflect on how you make meaning of the situation, by using the schema in Figure 3.2. Can you see where you might be conforming to behavioural norms and where meaning is coming from developing ideas and reflexive awareness?

There is an outline answer to this activity at the end of the chapter.

Having identified some brief experiences from your own life and how you develop meaning, and following on from what you have learned so far about autobiographical reflection and integrating personal and professional experiences, we now proceed to a life story exercise that helps you to prepare your autobiography.

Life story exercise – preparing your autobiography

Compile a written account of your life story so far. This might include aspects such as:

- where you were born;
- family and friends;
- growing up;
- significant events;
- school;
- first job;
- choice of career;
- interests.

Illustrate the aspects you have chosen to include with examples. In talking about specific events, try to focus on their meaning as well as their factual content. When you have completed the account, think about the following questions.

- Whose voices appear in the construction?
- How did constructing your autobiography make you feel?
- How do you regulate emotion?
- Did you have any concerns and, if so, what were these?
- Are there elements you wish to change and, if so, why?
- What might this process tell you about working with clients/patients?

This exercise might help you to develop self-awareness of your values and developing professional values. Having asked you to compile your own autobiography, we now proceed to considering how you might examine and reflect upon its content to develop your learning.

How to examine and reflect upon autobiography

You may have taken some time to decide what to put into your autobiography. Such decisions are likely to be influenced by what the purpose is in writing it, who the potential readers are and what range of experiences there are to choose from. All of these aspects are analytical points of interest when starting to examine your autobiography.

How the autobiography is structured can convey a sense of how you have been shaped by the events you have experienced and, at the same time, may also be a process of repair and change where experiences have been difficult or painful (Fischer-Rosenthal, 2000). Examining your autobiography is a tool for developing self-awareness and reflecting upon it is a way of being able to actively influence future direction and initiate change.

It takes considerable time, effort and emotional fortitude to properly examine and reflect on your autobiography. This starts from the time of assembling it and continues through to its completion and afterwards. Questions of context, feelings and knowledge base are an important feature in all types of reflection. However, when questioning autobiography these questions are inadequate on their own to gain sufficiently meaningful answers to what a personal life brings to the situation and to personal development. What is needed is also to focus upon the connections between experiences past, present and future, and to examine ways in which thinking is changing and personal responses to this. Other important aspects to consider include the regulation of emotion in terms of how it is portrayed, and examining different voices and emerging themes (Horsdal, 2012). This enables looking at what is being internalised and how this occurs.

The scenario of Libby's biographical account is provided to help illustrate some significant features that may be relevant to past, present and future learning and associated emotional aspects. You are asked to identify some of these features after reading the scenario.

Scenario: Libby's biographical account

Libby is in the first semester of her nurse preparation programme. She started the course in September after completing her 'A' levels in the summer. She is enjoying the challenge of the course and has made some good friends. She also enjoys the hustle and bustle of living in a city. She particularly enjoys the more independent mode of study when compared to school, where she had felt restricted to the teachers' thinking.

Libby comes from an army family and is the middle child of three. Her family circumstances meant moving home and school frequently. Libby got particularly upset when she had to leave her friend Natasha behind in year 9 and move to another school.

Libby's mother is a nurse and encouraged her daughter to go into nursing because of the transferability of the skills she will learn. Libby's family is currently located in Canada. To help develop other interests Libby has joined a local swimming club and helps out with the coaching when she can. She likes working with the

continued . . .

beginners the best. Libby misses her family and uses **Skype** *to keep in touch as often as she can. She has recently received her first assignment mark of 68 per cent and is keen to share this as soon as she can with her family, but has to wait due to the time difference. She finds this frustrating.*

Question

• What are the significant features within this biographical account and why?

There is an outline answer to this question at the end of the chapter.

Having read Libby's biographical account and answered the question at the end, you will be able to see that examining and reflecting are not the same. Examining your autobiography means collating events and looking for particular features. Examining your autobiography means paying attention to the factual content. This might include questions such as the following.

• What is the timeline of events? Identifying the timeline gives clues to the different stages of your life and how these might relate to external events.
• What decisions were made? Decision making can provide information about how you were thinking at the time.
• How is identity visible? Tracing the thread of an identity helps to raise awareness of changes and the circumstances that affect this.
• Where is learning evident? Identifying learning helps to develop personal knowledge.

Examining your autobiography also requires asking more contemplative questions about the relationships between people and the construction of the story. For example, what is underlying the direction and focus of the construction and its inclusions? This helps to then advance into reflection on more hidden meaning.

It is by reflecting upon your autobiographical account that sense can be made from it in distinguishing between then and now and how meaning is constantly evolving in the light of new knowledge, connections made, strategies identified and learning taken forward. Equally, reflecting upon the features within it also starts to reveal changes in your identity as you develop. Such development can be called a process of '**becoming**', as the novice professional grows in skill and knowledge of what it is to be a professional (Maich et al., 2000). Initially, reflecting might include the following questions.

• What from personal history gives this event significance? Looking across life experience and reviewing what is active in noticing is one way to start making the connections from which new insights emerge.
• What meaning does this have? Making sense of new insights requires defining what we mean.
• What did the surrounding context contribute to this meaning? Contexts encompass objects, people, cultures and society, all of which influence behaviour and the meaning given to something.
• How do I feel about this now? Reviewing changing feelings helps to acknowledge and make sense of emotional learning and associated developing thinking.

- How is my identity changing? Reviewing a changing identity helps to develop self-awareness and reflexivity in how events are shaping you as a person and a professional.

However, contemplative reflecting requires asking broader questions about the role we take in shaping our world and the role of the world in shaping us. For example, a person who has come from another country, or perhaps even just another region, will have an identity that is rooted in the cultural values of that place. The starting point is to reflect on what these might be in the first instance, in order to be able to identify a change and where that then stems from – whether from the person or a necessity to perhaps conform.

Now use these suggestions about examining and reflecting on your autobiography to complete Activity 3.5.

Activity 3.5   *Critical thinking*

Examine and reflect on your own autobiography, which you compiled earlier, using the suggestions above and the following questions.

- What might your autobiography contribute to your learning to be a professional?
- What potential alternative strategies does your autobiography contribute to your learning and decision making?
- What analytical conclusions have you reached from this exercise?
- What new insights have you developed and why?

There is an outline answer to this activity at the end of the chapter.

Having asked you to examine and reflect on your own autobiography, we now move on to consider how this relates to the perception of societal issues.

Identifying subjective perception of societal issues

Developing an autobiography can help to illustrate issues that are present in society by how they actually affect individuals through the lived experience of them. This is one way in which an autobiography raises awareness of social processes (West, 2001). In healthcare, the professional needs to be conscious of the uniqueness of each patient, but at the same time remain aware of how individual patient health experiences contribute to a wider understanding of health issues. For example, an experience of unemployment that you have had may reveal how welfare is organised and thought of within societal structures. Such experiences may even change your previously held views and social values, because of the power of the message imparted through your subjective experience, which may have far-reaching and lifelong effects. This can create a lens through which social issues and others' experiences become perceived.

Critically reflecting on subjective experience is one way not only to acknowledge its value in developing understanding, but also to reveal how personal views might have become shaped by others and entrenched as norms. What is perceived as normal and helpful through childhood experiences may be viewed very differently when looking back more critically from adult experience (Brookfield, 2005). Such critical reflection looks back and examines issues of power surrounding events and the learning taken from them. The following case study of subjective perception of societal issues provides an illustration of such a process.

Case study: identifying subjective perception of societal issues

Kelly is in the third year of her nurse preparation programme. In this year the focus of the modules she is undertaking is on developing skills in leadership and managing care, and on making the transition into practice. Kelly has had a recent placement within a surgical ward. She managed the care of a number of women. One in particular, Jane, has troubled her and she is trying to critically reflect on the situation, which has led her to question her own values and those of society.

Jane was admitted by Kelly for an excision breast biopsy for suspected breast cancer. Jane also had learning disabilities and so attended with her carer. Kelly is puzzled by this. She has a brother with learning disabilities and he has always lived with the family and gone to a mainstream school. Kelly starts to admit Jane by talking to her directly, but the carer intervenes, answering on her behalf. Kelly completes Jane's admission and starts to prepare her for the procedure. It is clear that Jane is frightened and confused by what is happening, so Kelly takes some time to sit with her and explain what she is doing. She uses her drawing skills to show Jane what she means when it is clear that Jane does not understand, and she does the same when the surgeon and anaesthetist come to see her. Kelly accompanies Jane to theatre and collects her as well to ensure that she sees a familiar face.

When reflecting on this incident there are a number of issues that come to the fore for Kelly. She sees the person, not the deficit. She has also noticed the limited response of the surgeon and anaesthetist when faced by Jane's incomprehension. She wonders whether the learning disabled service user's voice is heard by those aiming to care for them. When reflecting on her own experience Kelly realises that her own values and beliefs of seeing the person rather than a deficit are based on her experiences with her brother. She has assumed that these values are more mainstream because her brother's school friends accept him as he is.

Having seen the difficulty that there is within certain institutions, such as the hospital, she questions whether these difficulties also stem from a society that is less comfortable with difference and that therefore has not created appropriate provision according to person-centred need, but rather according to deficit. Kelly looks at why her values are different. She has grown up with her brother and knows him and his ways. Would she find his outbursts frightening if she did not know him? She wonders how much of this is related to control. Is a deficit model a kind of control? Kelly realises that control comes in many forms, not least in building relationships.

In this case study Kelly has identified disharmony between her taken-for-granted values and those she is experiencing in her student practitioner role. This has led her to reflect on why societal values might differ from hers and to question her assumptions. From such a position Kelly is able to advocate more effectively for her patient by entering into the societal debate more knowledgeably. Complete Activity 3.6 to identify some of your own values and assumptions.

Activity 3.6 — *Critical thinking*

Can you think of any experiences in your own life that helped to develop your understanding of some social issues? Reflect on these by looking at the following questions.

- What were the assumptions surrounding the situation?
- What values were active in the situation?
- What did you learn about the social issue?
- Has anything changed as a result of this learning?

There is an outline answer to this activity at the end of the chapter.

Having identified your own assumptions and values through the activity and by reflecting on the learning you have achieved in the situations you reflected on, you may potentially be able to be a more effective advocate for your patient in similar circumstances.

Chapter summary

This chapter has explained the ways in which autobiography can contribute to learning as a professional. By offering a number of suggestions of how to compile, examine and reflect on a personal biography, the chapter provided the starting and developing student nurse with the possibility of integrating personal and professional experiences into something meaningful to their learning. In this way it becomes possible to better understand personal learning needs and objectives and developing professional values, and to recognise a developing identity.

Activities and scenarios: Brief outline answers

Activity 3.1: Reflection (page 37)

The learning David is likely to have taken forward is:

- formal learning can be painful.

Reflective application

The meaning that David is likely to have attached is:

- he is not liked;
- he can sometimes teach others;
- asking for support is good.

Some creative strategies that David could employ might be:

- to focus on trying to articulate the subjects he needs to learn, as if he were teaching his friend;
- to harness his friend as a study buddy;
- to use his sense of drama to bring subjects to life;
- to talk things over with teachers.

Activity 3.2: Critical thinking (page 37)

Your answer might have related to the following key points:

- recognising important relationships;
- acknowledging emotional blocks and drivers in learning;
- developing understanding of strengths and areas of development;
- developing self-knowledge.

Activity 3.3: Reflection (page 38)

You might have expanded the list further to include:

- artist;
- activist;
- volunteer;
- carer.

The knowledge derived from the roles is dependent on time in the role, transferable skills and confidence.

Activity 3.4: Critical thinking (page 42)

When thinking about first starting the nurse preparation programme or moving into practice, you might have included:

- needing to identify what was expected by the regulatory body;
- professional behaviours;
- knowledge base.

When considering integrating thinking, you might have included:

- working interprofessionally to gain a wider perspective;
- reflecting on reasons for anxiety and uncertainty and addressing knowledge gaps;
- integrating reflective and imaginative ideas.

Activity 3.5: Critical thinking (page 45)

You might have addressed this activity by considering events about difficulty, how the past has been overcome, and how you are taking something forward into the future in a more positive way. Or you might have used a cautionary tale of how not to proceed, or a moral story of the right thing to do. Reflection may have included looking at emotional as well as cognitive learning, and how your identity is developing.

Activity 3.6: Critical thinking (page 47)

Answers to the activity are likely to have centred around:

- values such as dignity and respect, person-centredness and holistic care;
- assumptions;
- societal views;
- learning.

Scenario: David's biographical account of school (page 36)

See the answer to Activity 3.1 above.

Scenario: Libby's biographical account (pages 43–4)

This scenario includes the following features, which provide a good starting point for further examination and reflection on what is brought to the nursing course and how this is progressing:

*   moving schools and changing study experiences;
*   enjoying social processes;
*   family moving;
*   loss of best friend;
*   teaching and leadership skills;
*   struggle with missing family;
*   self-reliance.

Further reading

Dominice, P (2000) *Learning from Ourselves.* San Francisco, CA: Jossey-Bass.

This book identifies how preparing an educational biography can help with understanding processes of learning.

Horsdal, M (2012) *Telling Lives: Exploring dimensions of narratives.* Abingdon: Routledge.

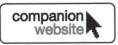

For further activities and other useful material, visit the companion website at
www.sagepub.co.uk/howatson-jones_reflective2e

Chapter 4
Reflective models and frameworks

NMC Standards for Pre-registration Nursing Education

This chapter will address the following competency:

Domain 4: Leadership, management and team working

2. All nurses must systematically evaluate care and ensure that they and others use the findings to help improve people's experience and care outcomes and to shape future services.

NMC Essential Skills Clusters

This chapter will address the following ESCs:

6. People can trust the newly registered graduate nurse to engage therapeutically and actively listen to their needs and concerns, responding using skills that are helpful, providing information that is clear, accurate, meaningful and free from jargon.

By the first progression point:

1. Communicates effectively both orally and in writing, so that the meaning is always clear.

By the second progression point:

6. Uses strategies to enhance communication and remove barriers to effective communication, minimising risk to people from lack of or poor communication.

Chapter aims

After reading this chapter you will be able to:

- identify different models and frameworks of reflection;
- consider strengths and limitations of different models and frameworks;
- choose an appropriate model or framework for your reflection.

Example story

Holly was working in an outpatient department in the second year of her nurse preparation programme. The consultant informed an 18-year-old girl, Maria, that her test results confirmed that she had leukaemia, and would need to have some treatment organised. He explained what the treatment would involve rapidly, then asked Holly's mentor to take Maria to another room to await another, more junior, doctor to organise this. This made Holly really angry because she did not think this was the way to tell someone such bad news. Maria had nobody with her. Surely, it would have been better to invite a family member in to be with her, but Holly thought this might have created problems with confidentiality. The consultant could at least have asked Maria if she wanted someone there. Holly felt the consultant's behaviour was very uncaring, and Holly's mentor had had to leave her with Maria because she had to go with the consultant to see another patient. Holly did not know what to do or say, although she had previously spoken to Maria in the waiting room because they were quite similar in age. Holly was shocked because she did not expect to see someone so young become seriously ill. If Maria had cried it might have been easier for Holly to know what to do, because this would have been a clear signal of distress. But Maria did not look distressed; she just plugged her iPod earphones into her ears and sat down. Holly had read about people's reactions to bad news and how varied they can be.

Looking back, Holly wondered whether Maria's behaviour could be interpreted as a sign of denial, of trying to block out what she had just been told. So what had Holly's choices been? Holly thought she could have sat by Maria to indicate her willingness to listen, and that she was there for her, perhaps using light touch to communicate her empathy. Holly had been told by her mentor that this could be very therapeutic, but must be used with caution. Holly could have offered to call a member of Maria's family. Or she could have given Maria verbal permission to cry, saying it was all right and might help, because Maria might have felt that this was not acceptable. However, Holly would also have needed to consider Maria's possible reactions to her. Maria might have related to Holly because of their similarity in age, but equally this might have made her resentful of Holly's apparent health. Holly also needed to be aware of the impact on herself with regard to the reality of potential illness at any age, including hers.

Holly's mentor came back and took over, sending Holly for a break. When she came back, Maria had gone to CT. Holly left the department at the end of the day feeling very frustrated and dissatisfied with Maria's care.

Holly thought about what she might have done differently. She could have sat with Maria to give her the opportunity to open up and take her cue from her. If Holly felt out of her depth, she would have been honest with Maria and acknowledged this, but called another member of staff to help. Holly would also read more about communication, particularly in relation to the breaking of bad news. Holly decided to discuss this issue further with her mentor to see what else she might have done, or how it could have been handled differently.

Introduction

The example offered above demonstrates how difficult situations, as well as those that arouse emotions, can stimulate thinking about them. The example will be reworked further through a **reflective cycle**, to help demonstrate some of the different stages of a reflective process. Using models and reflective cycles can help you, especially if you are less experienced, to develop your reflection into something that enables you to really examine your learning.

This chapter will introduce some of the wide range of reflective models and frameworks on which you can draw when first starting to structure and frame your reflections. You will be encouraged to consider some of the strengths and limitations of the selected reflective frameworks, models and cycles, to help you to choose appropriately. The right questions to ask will also be highlighted through the example and case study presented.

Reflective frameworks

Donald Schön (1991) examined how professionals think about what they are doing and described these ways of thinking as reflection-in-action and reflection-on-action. When in a situation, we are constantly reworking problems and discovering consequences from this reworking, and these have implications for further adaptations. Schön (1991) identifies this as a framing process whereby, through reframing roles and perspectives of a situation, new phenomena come into view and can be worked in other ways that may bring different solutions. Reflection-in-action can, therefore, be described as a form of experimentation in problem solving that acknowledges uncertainty and looks at discovering potential answers or ways to proceed. Schön (1991, p76) describes this as having a *reflective conversation with the situation*, which is also the strength of this approach, in that it is working with the situation in real time. In other words, we are constantly interpreting and responding to cues within the situation and consequently changing its course in the process. Nevertheless, a limitation is that much of this reflection often occurs unconsciously as part of working with experience intuitively. 'Intuitively' means that articulated descriptions can never fully explain the actions taken or knowledge used, or *artistry* involved (Schön, 1991, p276). Undertaking Activity 4.1 will help you to understand these points.

Activity 4.1   *Evidence-based practice and research*

Observe someone undertaking an activity. It might be your mentor in practice or a teacher in class. If you are an experienced practitioner it might be an advanced practitioner in their field. Consider how their activity flows and whether they seem to be aware of each process or step they are undertaking. For example, think about the following.

- When is it obvious to you that they have in some way modified their actions?
- Were there hesitations when they might have thought about what they were doing and altered direction?

---

continued . . .

- What happened when you, or somebody else, asked them a question?
- How was the answer worked out?

There is an outline answer to this activity at the end of the chapter.

The process of reflection-in-action is the experiential part that enables adaptation of learning from experience during action. Critical analysis, which will be explored in the guise of critical reflection in more detail in Chapter 11, helps to formalise and record these processes. When completing nursing activities yourself, you may have become aware that you are not conscious of thoughts at the time but that you are responding to what the situation might require. This is because, when we stop, we become more aware of what is going on in our thinking as well as acting. We also become conscious of what we have learned through the action we have undertaken, when looking back on it. Schön (1991) suggests that thinking too much about action when undertaking it might raise barriers to the smooth flow of action. This, therefore, may become a limitation. However, looking back at action can help the professional to gain greater insight and clarity in their thought processes and the actions taken. This is called reflection-on-action. The process of reflection-on-action highlights the learning achieved for future use and is particularly useful for the novice to undertake. Completing Activity 4.2 may help you to identify some of your own learning from reflection-on-action.

Activity 4.2   *Critical thinking*

Think of a time recently when you worked with your mentor. If you are an experienced practitioner, think of a time when you worked with a student. Consider a patient problem that you dealt with together.

- What was the patient problem?
- Was the problem clear to you both at the start?
- Were there different interpretations of the problem during the situation?
- How did this become clear?
- Were you conscious of this during the situation?
- What discoveries did you make during the situation?
- How did these influence your further actions?
- How did your further actions act on the problem?
- What learning are you taking away from the situation?

There is an outline answer to this activity at the end of the chapter.

As you completed Activity 4.2 you might have become aware of other aspects that were not obvious to you at the time of the event. You may also have identified gaps in your knowledge. We proceed now to consider how using a reflective model can help you to question some of these elements in order to develop your learning.

Reflective models

Reflection requires effort of attentive consideration to thoughts and feelings and memories to make appropriate changes (Taylor, 2010, p6). For example, you might identify that you find it emotionally difficult when dealing with death and dying. Using a model helps you to identify key stages of your reflective learning and the structure can help you to keep going when you are dealing with complex issues, in order to arrive at some resolution as to how to deal with situations. It is important to choose a model that suits your needs and that you find easy to use. Nevertheless, for reflection to be of value and to maintain progression of your lifelong learning, it is important to reflect on what you are doing and on your learning regularly, and for reflection to become embedded as a part of who you are as a learner and practitioner. The following models offer a number of perspectives on areas to focus your reflection on and questions you might want to ask yourself. Johns has developed and refined the following model over a number of years and through working with many practitioners at different stages of their development (Johns, 1995, 1997, 2002). This is an important point to realise: reflection is dynamic and the ways in which it is undertaken are constantly evolving. Therefore, any model can only ever be a guide rather than an ending in itself.

Model for Structured Reflection

The Model for Structured Reflection (MSR) (Johns, 2004) identifies how you might want to examine your experience more extensively and in greater depth in order to really learn from it. The model's starting point is to create space for reflection – what Johns (2004) calls *bringing the mind home*, which means stilling the mind so it can focus. The model then encompasses a number of reflective cues, or questions, which the practitioner is asked to think about in the course of reflecting on a situation. These are presented below.

Concept summary: MSR reflective cues

- Bringing the mind home.
- Description.
- Reflection on what occurred in terms of the following.
  - How was I feeling and what made me feel that way?
  - What was I trying to achieve?
  - Did I respond effectively?
  - What were the consequences of my actions for the patient, others and myself?
  - How were others feeling, and what made them feel that way?
  - What factors influenced the way I was feeling, thinking or responding?
  - What knowledge might have informed me?
  - To what extent did I act for the best and in tune with my values?
- Alternatives.
  - How does this situation connect with previous experiences?
  - How might I respond more effectively given this situation again?

> – What would be the consequences of alternative actions for the patient, others and myself?
> - Changes.
>   – How do I now feel about this experience?
>   – Am I now more able to support myself and others better as a consequence?
>
> (Source: Johns, Christopher (2004) *Becoming a Reflective Practitioner: A reflective and holistic approach to clinical nursing, practice development and clinical supervision*, pp20–7. © 2004 Blackwell Science Publishing Ltd. Reproduced with written permission of Blackwell Science Publishing Ltd.)

These cues encompass aesthetic, personal, ethical, empirical and reflexive aspects that are related to Carper's (1978) fundamental patterns of knowing (Johns, 1995).

- Aesthetics relates to how the person feels about, responds to and perceives the situation and those involved.
- Personal aspects explore what from the person was influencing them.
- Ethics encompasses how actions are related to beliefs.
- Empirics is concerned with what knowledge was used.
- Reflexivity relates to how experiences are connected and the possible alternatives and changes to doing things differently.

The following case study makes use of these cues in order to help illustrate how this model might be applied.

Case study: Tamara's experience of comforting

Tamara was working on a gynaecology ward and her mentor had arranged for her to spend some time in the Early Pregnancy Unit with the scanning nurse, Pip. Pip scanned a lady called Jane and found that there was no fetal heartbeat. When she informed Jane of this she was understandably very upset. Pip asked Tamara to stay with Jane while she made further arrangements.

Tamara took Jane somewhere quiet where they could talk in private. She thought that Jane would probably want to be away from prying eyes. Tamara began by saying how sorry she was and that it was all right for Jane to express her feelings. Jane began to cry quietly. Tamara sat close to her, but not touching, as she was not sure how Jane would react to a stranger as she did not like strangers touching her. She allowed Jane to cry for a while and then asked her if she wanted anyone to be contacted. Jane said her partner was at work and she did not want to disturb him. She asked why the miscarriage had happened. Tamara explained that she was a student nurse and would get Pip. At that moment Pip came into the room to explain the next steps. She told Jane that the reasons for miscarriage are often not known, although further tests would be carried out. Both Pip and Jane thanked Tamara for being there.

continued . . .

Later that day Tamara's link tutor, Lynne, came to the ward. She could see that Tamara looked upset so she took her to a quiet area to talk. Tamara told Lynne about her morning and how it had upset her. She felt that she should have done more, but was not sure what she could have done. Lynne helped Tamara to reflect on the situation. They identified that Tamara had used a person-centred approach by offering Jane privacy and giving her time to express her feelings. Tamara had not imposed her own views of the situation and had sought help when asked questions that were outside her sphere of knowledge. Lynne asked Tamara what she had learned from the situation. Tamara said that the overriding thing she had learned was that we do not always have answers. She felt she could perhaps have done more in comforting Jane. Lynne and Tamara explored the options of using touch. Lynne advised Tamara to revisit communication literature. Tamara felt less upset and thought that, next time, she would talk to her mentor about the situation. Nevertheless, she felt she had handled a difficult situation well.

The case study illustrates how reflection can also affirm actions as well as correct them. Using this model helps to surface how others might also be thinking and how to deal with it.

Stages of reflection

We move on now to consider another model by Atkins and Murphy (1995), which examines three main stages to reflection based on feelings, knowledge and coming to new ways of thinking.

- Stage 1 – Awareness of uncomfortable feelings.
- Stage 2 – Critical analysis of the situation.
- Stage 3 – Development of new perspectives on the situation.

(Taken from Atkins, S and Murphy, K (1995) Reflective practice. *Nursing Standard*, 9(45), August. Used by kind permission of RCN Publishing Co. Ltd.)

Stage 1 of this model relates to uncomfortable feelings being the stimulus for starting to reflect on what is causing them and what can be done. Part of this will be an assessment of your knowledge base and whether this was sufficient. Atkins and Murphy (1995) make the point here that feelings need not necessarily be negative, but can be more positively related to some achievement. It might be useful to qualify this point with reference to Jarvis (2007, p3) who describes such a state as 'disharmony', which occurs when there is a break with familiar experience that alerts the person reflecting to a change taking place. Stage 2 relates to examining the use of knowledge and potential gaps in knowledge as well as the effects on the individual and the situation and how the individual affected this. The purpose here is to connect feelings, knowledge and information with the situation and the individual so that the person is able to develop new insights. Stage 3 clarifies what these insights are by describing them as 'outcomes of reflection' and how this learning will be taken forward (Atkins and Murphy, 1995, p2).

Model of reflection from a student's perspective

Another model that you might find useful is Stephenson's (1993) model, which looks at reflection from the student's perspective. This is based on students questioning their roles, feelings, actions, expectations and knowledge, as well as some of the broader surrounding issues within which their experiences may be embedded. These questions are extremely relevant to your stage of learning and are particularly helpful by asking you to relate your professional practice to the wider political and social world, which may exert influence over what is happening and what you can do.

The main questions of Stephenson's (1993) model are as follows.

Concept summary: Stephenson's model of reflection (from a student's perspective)

- What was my role in the situation?
- Did I feel comfortable or uncomfortable? Why?
- What actions did I take?
- How did I and others act?
- Was it appropriate?
- How could I have improved the situation for myself, the patient, my mentor?
- How can I change in future?
- Do I feel as if I have learnt anything new about myself?
- Did I expect anything different to happen? What and why?
- Has it changed my way of thinking in any way?
- What knowledge from theory and research can I apply to this situation?
- What broader issues, for example political or social, arise from this situation?
- What do I think about these broader issues?

(Source: Stephenson (1993), cited in Palmer, A, Burns, S and Bulman, C (1994) *Reflective Practice in Nursing: The growth of the Professional Practitioner*, p137. © 1994 Blackwell Science Publishing Ltd. Reproduced with permission of Blackwell Science Publishing Ltd.)

The more experienced practitioner might want to use these questions with students as a part of the teaching and assessing process to develop reflective learning together.

The final model offered by Howatson-Jones (2010) suggests some exploratory questions that are meant to stimulate reflective thinking from a broader historical sense. These stem from personal research and are particularly relevant to reflections about working with people.

Concept summary: A biographical perspective on reflection

- What foreknowledge did I bring to the situation and what do I need to know?
- What action did I take in the situation and why?
- How might others' perceptions be framing their responses?
- What is the quality of the response and how does it make me feel and act?
- What connections are there between responses now and earlier?
- Are there contraindications? Why?

- What from autobiography is influencing my noticing?
- What other factors might be influencing the situation?
- What does the language used in, or about, the situation reveal?
- What dimensions does my learning take, for example psychological, physiological, affective (behavioural), spiritual, biographical?

(Source: Howatson-Jones (2010).)

The questions offered above provide an opportunity to reflect on how your biography can be active in what you notice and how you might reflect. This is an important point to question to ensure that blind spots do not develop, as these can hinder the ability to respond in better ways. Equally, developing biographical understanding can help you to read situations in different ways, such as how particular arenas of nursing work and why certain units have issues with others. The term 'model' is sometimes used interchangeably with the term 'reflective cycle'. In essence, both offer structure to help you to examine your reflective learning. Some, however, are more cyclical and are therefore referred to as reflective cycles. We proceed now to explore some reflective cycles.

Reflective cycles

Reflective cycles offer the possibility to connect what has been learned from one experience with that of another. Using a reflective cycle can help you to clarify how your learning is progressing and what you need to do to support it further, and enables you to plan further action and set objectives relating to this. There are a number of different reflective cycles that you can choose from and use. One of the most well-known reflective cycles is that of Gibbs (1988), which outlines specific steps to guide the learner through processes of description, acknowledgement of feelings, evaluation, analysis and action planning, as outlined in Figure 4.1.

The description of the situation is limited to the salient points, which are the main priorities. By acknowledging feelings, the learner is able to consider processes, such as how to deal with sometimes difficult emotions that may be aroused by caring work and learning. Evaluation begins to think about what are the main issues. These can then be analysed in greater detail by considering what knowledge is available, or might need to be developed, and what other choices might have been accessible in the situation and the possible consequences if one of those choices had been chosen instead. From this analysis follows consideration of changes to thinking about this type of situation and how maybe to proceed the next time. From here, further action is then planned. The important aspects of this cycle are that analysis should result in some kind of action planning to take learning forward.

Now apply Gibbs' reflective cycle to the 'Example story' provided at the start of the chapter by completing Activity 4.3.

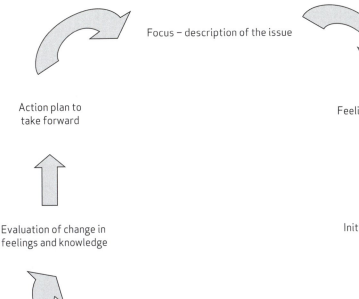

Focus – description of the issue

Feelings produced

Action plan to
take forward

Initial evaluation

Evaluation of change in
feelings and knowledge

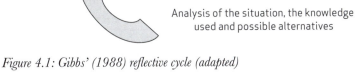

Analysis of the situation, the knowledge
used and possible alternatives

Figure 4.1: Gibbs' (1988) reflective cycle (adapted)
(Used with kind permission of OCSLD: Oxford Brookes University.)

Activity 4.3   *Communication*

- Using the key stages of Gibbs' (1988) reflective cycle, identify which parts of the example fit with these key stages. It might help to write these out on a separate piece of paper.
- Now underline the actual words within the parts of the example which represent the action points of the key stages of the reflective cycle which you have placed them under.

There is an outline answer to this activity at the end of the chapter.

From applying Gibbs' (1988) reflective cycle to the example at the start of the chapter, you might have identified that Holly needed to learn more about the processes of breaking bad news in order to be able to challenge less effective practice and develop her own communication skills. A developed cycle based on Gibbs can be found in the Davis model, which includes an additional stage of considering the evidence base for change (Davis et al., 2011). You are directed to the book *Learning Skills for Nursing Students* (Davis et al., 2011), also in this series, to learn more. We proceed now to look at a different reflective cycle.

Driscoll's (2007, p44) reflective cycle has its roots in experiential learning and views reflection as a process of interrogating.

- What?
- So what?
- Now what?

These three questions encompass the need to be clear in the interpretation, interrogation and presentation of learning through reflection. The 'what?' refers to being able to describe the situation in words. This requires some mental ordering of events and helps to start the reflective process. The 'so what?' involves beginning to analyse important aspects of the experience from which new discoveries may appear. The 'now what?' proposes new actions based on these discoveries and which may be reworked in multiple different situations. Driscoll's cycle (2007) is simple, but effective. It is easy to remember and these questions can easily be asked as part of most conversations within the classroom or practice and, therefore, can multiply the opportunities for reflection.

You may have noticed some similarities between the various frameworks, models and cycles of reflection. The next cycle acknowledges this point and is founded on the main principles we have looked at so far.

Jasper (2003, p2) suggests that most cycles of reflection are founded on the principles of experience-reflection-action (ERA). The reflective cycle starts with some kind of experience or situation in which you are, or have been, involved. Experience may be something recent or something that you have developed. Reflection relates to reviewing and looking at the familiar as well as the unfamiliar with fresh eyes, in order to consider what resources are available to you, who is, or needs to be, involved and what other strategies are available to you. Action refers to the implementation of learning and new strategies. These cycles of reflection may spiral one to another over a period of time (Jasper, 2003) forming part of a process of becoming as the person develops themselves and their knowledge (Johns, 2009). In other words, by connecting learning from different reflective episodes, you will be in a better position to get a clearer view of how you are developing your knowledge of yourself, your profession, your environment and culture and of other people, as well as the theoretical knowledge that underpins this. Reflection is about being able to connect experience with what you do.

Having looked at a number of different **reflective frameworks**, models and cycles, complete Activity 4.4 in order to clarify your understanding of them.

Activity 4.4 — *Critical thinking*

- What are the main commonalities and differences between the various frameworks, models and cycles?
- Which of them appear easier to use and why?
- Which of them appear harder to use and why?
- Are there different types of situations that the different frameworks, models and cycles are suited to? If so, why?
- What do you see as the strengths and limitations of each of the frameworks, models and cycles?

There is an outline answer to this activity at the end of the chapter.

> ## Chapter summary
>
> This chapter has introduced and explored a number of different reflective frameworks, models and cycles that you can choose from when starting or continuing to reflect.
>
> Through the example story, case study and activities provided you have been given the opportunity to apply a variety of reflective formats. These are not an end in themselves but offer you a starting point from which to develop your own reflective journey. Nevertheless, they assist with structuring what might sometimes be painful and difficult to admit to yourself, as well as help you to identify how to replicate and multiply successes. When time is short, the discipline of a reflective framework can help to keep you on track. How to create space for such reflection is explored in greater depth in the next chapter.

Activities: Brief outline answers

Activity 4.1: Evidence-based practice and research (pages 52–3)

You might have observed that your mentor, teacher or advanced practitioner was able to talk around the subject effortlessly while undertaking the tasks of practice or teaching. You might, for example, have noted your mentor adjusting a wound dressing technique in response to the patient wincing, all the while telling them what the wound dressing was for and how it was progressing. Similarly, you might have been in a clinical science class and observed the teacher responding to some people's confusion by asking class members to take on the role of oxygen and sit in a haemoglobin 'car' made up of four chairs that could take four passengers. You might have observed the advanced practitioner skilfully completing an examination while teaching the patient and you. There might have been a fleeting hesitation while the mentor, teacher or advanced practitioner took in the cues they received from the patient/class, but the alteration in what they did next would have been imperceptible. However, if the patient asks a question of the mentor and a student asks the teacher, there is a more perceptible pause to think of the answer to give. The answer is likely to have involved some dialogue to check whether it met the expectation of the questioner and that they also understood the answer.

Activity 4.2: Critical thinking (page 53)

You might have considered a patient problem relating to developing a pressure sore. You and your mentor or your student may have noted a change in skin colour and appearance. There may have been a difference in interpretation of the severity of the problem due to difference in knowledge. You may not have realised this until comparing the scores you took, and you might have discovered that, when using some scoring systems, it is easy to overestimate risk. You might have been surprised by the degree of subjectivity still involved. If you are an experienced practitioner you might have considered your accountability should the patient develop a pressure sore. You might have been more careful to regularly assess the risk using the same tool each time to monitor changes. You may have learned that assessment tools are only as good as the knowledge and observation of the person using them.

Activity 4.3: Communication (page 59)

Description

Holly was working in an outpatient department in the second year of her nurse preparation programme. The consultant informed an 18-year-old girl, Maria, that her test results confirmed that she had leukaemia, and would need to have some treatment organised. He explained what the treatment would involve rapidly and then asked Holly's mentor to take Maria to another room to await another more junior doctor to organise this.

Feelings

This made Holly really angry because she did not think this was the way to tell someone such bad news. Maria had nobody with her.

Evaluation

Surely, it would have been better to invite a family member in to be with her, but Holly thought this might have created problems with confidentiality. The consultant could at least have asked Maria if she wanted someone to be there. Holly felt the consultant's behaviour was very uncaring, and Holly's mentor had had to leave her with Maria because she had to go with the consultant to see another patient. Holly did not know what to do or say, although she had previously spoken to Maria in the waiting room because they were quite similar in age. Holly was shocked because she did not expect to see someone so young become seriously ill. If Maria had cried it might have been easier for Holly to know what to do, because this would have been a clear signal of distress. But Maria did not look distressed; she just plugged her iPod earphones into her ears and sat down. Holly had read about people's reactions to bad news and how varied they can be.

Analysis

Looking back now, Holly wondered whether Maria's behaviour could be interpreted as a sign of denial, of trying to block out what she had just been told. So what had Holly's choices been? Holly thought she could have sat by Maria to indicate her willingness to listen, and that she was there for her, perhaps using light touch to communicate her empathy. Holly had been told by her mentor that this could be very therapeutic, but must be used with caution. Holly could have offered to call a member of Maria's family. Or she could have given Maria verbal permission to cry, saying it was all right and might help, because Maria might have felt that this was not acceptable. However, Holly would also have needed to consider Maria's possible reactions to her. Maria might have related to Holly because of their similarity in age, but equally this might have made her resentful of Holly's apparent health. Holly also needed to be aware of the impact on herself with regard to the reality of potential illness at any age, including hers. Holly's mentor came back and took over, sending Holly for a break. When she came back, Maria had gone to CT. Holly left the department at the end of the day feeling very frustrated and dissatisfied with Maria's care.

Evaluation of change

Holly thought about what she might have done differently. She could have sat with Maria to give her the opportunity to open up and take her cue from her. If Holly felt out of her depth, she would have been honest with Maria and acknowledged this, but called another member of staff to help.

Action planning

Holly would also read more about communication, particularly in relation to the breaking of bad news. Holly decided to discuss this issue further with her mentor to see what else she might have done, or how the situation could have been handled differently.

Activity 4.4: Critical thinking (page 60)

- You are likely to have identified that the areas of commonality between the different reflective formats include evaluation, analysis and action. Areas of difference might be, for you, in the depth of reflection demanded by the models in comparison to the easier application of the reflective cycles. The biographical model is also different in asking you to identify what is active in your noticing.

- You may have found reflection-in-action particularly relevant to starting to develop your practice skills, while reflection-on-action may have helped you to embed them. The reflective cycles might have helped you to structure reflection within assignments and when talking about practice. The models of reflection might have helped you to examine your learning in more detail through reflective writing.
- You are likely to have identified problem solving as a strength of reflection-in-action, while limited consciousness of the learning achieved might have been a limitation. Similarly, too much thought might be a barrier to developing reflection-on-action into action. You may have considered the potential depth for reflection as a strength of the models of reflection, but the time needed for this as a limitation. You may also have viewed the acknowledgement of feelings in some of the models and reflective cycles as a strength that helps to take feelings forward in more positive ways, but the simplicity of the reflective cycles might also encourage superficial examination of issues. You may have noticed that the biographical approach helped you to integrate your reflective learning better, but that this might also have been challenging in what you found out about yourself. You might also have thought about the importance of credible evidence on which to base changing practice.

Further reading

Bulman, C and **Schutz, S** (eds) (2008) *Reflective Practice in Nursing*, 4th edition. Oxford: Blackwell Scientific Publications.

Johns, C (2009) *Becoming a Reflective Practitioner*, 3rd edition. Chichester: Blackwell.

Taylor, B (2010) *Reflective Practice for Healthcare Professionals*, 3rd edition. Maidenhead: Open University Press.

These books offer in-depth explanations of some of the models and frameworks discussed in this chapter.

Davis, N, Clark, AC, O'Brien, M, Sumpton, K and Waugh, S (2011) *Learning Skills for Nursing Students*. Exeter: Learning Matters.

This book identifies reflection as a core graduate skill and shows how it links with all the other graduate skills students need to learn.

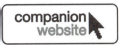 For further activities and other useful material, visit the companion website at **www.sagepub.co.uk/howatson-jones_reflective2e**

Chapter 5
Creating space for reflection

continued . . .

By the first progression point:

1. Works within the code (NMC 2008) and adheres to the *Guidance on professional conduct for nursing and midwifery students.* (NMC 2010).

By the second progression point:

2. Supports and assists others appropriately.
3. Values others' roles and responsibilities within the team and interacts appropriately.

Chapter aims

After reading this chapter you will be able to:

- define the concept of transitional space;
- identify some barriers and limitations to reflection and strategies for overcoming these;
- examine the kinds of relationships that exist between people and how these might be more caring and compassionate;
- consider how you negotiate your position within healthcare;
- identify what makes spaces compelling for reflection and learning.

Example story

Jamie was in the last year of his nurse preparation programme and was working on a medical ward. He had been assigned to work with another student nurse called Mariamma for the morning and was responsible for organising the care of eight patients in a bay. Jamie was developing his leadership and management skills as part of his transition into practice, and his mentor thought that working with another student would benefit them both. Mariamma was very nervous as this was only her second placement and everything still felt very new to her. She confided this to Jamie, who smilingly reassured her that he had felt the same way at the beginning of the programme. Jamie asked Mariamma if she knew how to complete the tasks that he delegated to her and kept an eye on her to be sure. Mariamma noticed that one of the patients was quite confused and that Jamie would, every so often between his organisational tasks, take time to talk to the patient and reassure him. As the morning progressed she realised that Jamie had a good rapport with most of the patients and that they responded to him warmly, Mariamma wondered whether she would ever be able to be like that.

Before handover at lunchtime Jamie asked Mariamma to help him to reflect briefly on the morning's work to ensure that all the relevant information was covered. During this discussion it seemed that both Jamie and Mariamma provided each other with feedback.

Mariamma asked Jamie how he had managed to develop such a good relationship with the patients. Jamie stopped for a moment to consider this and said he was not sure. Mariamma told him what she had observed in that Jamie appeared to approach the patients with a joke and smile at the ready. With the confused patient he toned this down, using a quieter voice and clear instructions. Jamie had not really thought about how he communicated and for him this was a bit of a revelation. He told Mariamma this and how helpful he had found working with her because of the opportunity it gave him to explain what he was doing and why. This helped him to clarify his knowledge and prioritise the information the next shift would need.

Jamie went into the handover feeling confident. He was fluent in what he was saying and left the shift feeling happy with a job well done. On his way home Jamie analysed why this might be and identified that having his actions affirmed and being able to demonstrate his knowledge were what were making him feel good. He considered that he might have used some of these communication techniques to help build up Mariamma's confidence and decided he would pay more attention to her as well as the patients next time.

Introduction

The example above helps to illustrate how nurses are able to collaborate and share in learning, creating space for reflection within other activity. Finding the time or a suitable place for reflection can be difficult. Often it is easy to find other things to put in its place, maybe because what reflection reveals makes you feel uncomfortable. Yet it is precisely continuing with familiar and comfortable ways of thinking and doing things that keeps you from exploring alternatives and considering change. Transition means moving from one position, or point of view, to another and represents the shift in between that can feel uncomfortable and uncertain. As you progress through your nurse preparation programme, or even your career, more is expected from you in terms of knowledge, skills and decision making.

This chapter will introduce the concept of reflection as a **transitional space** in which you are encouraged to explore, develop and grow. The chapter considers some of the barriers and limitations to reflection and strategies you can use to overcome these. The chapter will ask you to examine the relationships that exist between individuals and how you negotiate your place in diverse healthcare settings and situations. Finally, the chapter will explore care and compassion for oneself and others, and what makes spaces compelling for reflection and learning.

Finding the time and space for reflection

Finding the time and space for reflection requires interest, motivation and commitment, as has been discussed in the previous chapters. Taylor (2010) suggests that reflection should be undertaken daily. Making reflection a part of your routine means that you are more likely to continue with it and be able to see trends and changes taking place in both your practice and learning. This view suggests that, just as in the example above, space for reflection can be found within the activities of daily practice. However, such spaces frequently appear at the margins of activity and are necessarily often brief and hurried in terms of the time used. Consider the following scenario to help you to identify where such spaces might appear in both personal and professional life.

Scenario: Brett's day with the community mental health nurse

Brett was in the second year of his mental health nurse preparation programme. He was used to the inpatient environment and was now keen to extend his scope of practice by experiencing the community setting. He was due to visit a new patient, Keith, today with his mentor Mohammed. Brett woke at 6 a.m. although he did not need to be at work until 8 a.m. He had breakfast alone listening to the early news on the radio and then cycled the 15 minutes to work. Mohammed, his mentor, talked the initial assessment process over with Brett as they travelled in his car to visit Keith. Brett observed Mohammed undertaking the assessment and talked a little with Keith while Mohammed was writing. While Mohammed was fetching something from the car Keith told Brett that he felt very depressed and had considered suicide, but his family had so far stopped him carrying it out. He had a young son and he wanted desperately to get better for him so he could take him out. Brett and Mohammed left Keith's house and there was little time to discuss his situation as Mohammed was preparing Brett for their next visit of the day. At lunchtime Mohammed had an urgent errand in town and Brett went with him as he needed some money from the bank. They relaxed on the drive to town, talking about their shared interest in football. The afternoon passed in a blur with more visits and assessments. Brett cycled home feeling exhausted at the end of the day. When he got home he did half an hour of fitness, then shared a beer with his housemates over supper and finished an assignment before going to bed.

Question
- Which activities, or spaces between them, in this scenario offered possibilities for reflection?

There is an outline answer to this question at the end of the chapter.

Through this scenario you may have identified that there is scope and space for reflection, but that it is a person's focus, willingness and commitment to reflect that might be lacking. When time is limited, other priorities start to take over and it becomes difficult to maintain the discipline required for reflecting on your own learning in different situations inside and outside the classroom and in practice.

One way to help maintain reflection is to use supporting elements, such as reflecting with others, either in groups or choosing a critical friend, who can help to invite commitment and provide additional support (Bulman and Schutz, 2008). Such support makes it easier to face and deal with the changes that reflection inevitably brings. Peer support is an important part of reflection in that it offers the opportunity for a two-way process of learning from the dialogue (Johns, 2007). Such dialogue involves reflective telling as well as reflective receiving. For example, when discussing how you feel with someone else they are likely to ask you what sparked that emotion, which will stimulate you to reflect on some of the surrounding reasons and issues. Equally, your listener may then think about your reasoning and offer some of their own after reflecting on what you have said. In this way, reflection is mutually beneficial.

For the more experienced practitioner it is suggested that recognising practice to be complex, constantly evolving and full of surprises means that it is essential for self-reflection to be a part of everyday practice (Crabtree, 2003). Therefore, peer-reflective dialogue needs to be recognised as a normal part of professional practice. We proceed now to consider the kind of space created by the act of reflection.

Transitional space

Transitional space is, as the name suggests, a place where a person is in the throes of change. Jarvis (2006) identifies that learning means people move from a position of being to one of becoming. This means that, in the process of such adjustment, a person enters into a transitional space where there are a number of possibilities for their development that need to be negotiated, and where they may become changed as people. For example, you will have entered your nurse preparation programme with an idea of who you are, but during the course this may start to shift as you 'become' a nurse. Similarly, if you are an experienced practitioner you will have an idea of the kind of practitioner you are. Nevertheless, as you gather experience you will 'become' more expert, maybe a leader, or take another path such as becoming a nurse educator!

Transitional space, originally conceptualised by Winnicott (1965), is also defined as the point where subjective inner experience interacts with objective outer experience (Hunt and West, 2007) – in other words, the meaning we make of the external situations in which we find ourselves and that influence our development. The transitional space of learning is framed by how organisations and individuals that help to create such a space perceive themselves and interact. The following case study is provided as an example to help illustrate these processes.

Case study: Ellen's experience of failure

Ellen was at the end of the first year of her nurse preparation programme and had recently received exam results that required her to retake the exam. The classes had been difficult to concentrate on, and Ellen acknowledged that she did not like the subject of clinical science. She had done well with her other subjects and was a good communicator.

continued . . .

Ellen was devastated as she felt she had worked really hard. There was very limited feedback to guide her about where she had gone wrong. Her first thought was that too much was expected of the student. She also felt angry towards the tutor, who she felt had not explained things well enough. Ellen was tempted to quit the programme as this felt so impossible. Gradually, as her anger and emotional response subsided, Ellen started thinking about what she could do. Her friend Mitch, who had passed the exam, told her she would be mad to quit now as she had almost passed the first year. He offered to help Ellen with her revising.

When Mitch and Ellen were revising it became obvious that Ellen had focused on a number of body systems in too much depth and had not revised towards the learning outcomes for the module. Her knowledge of those particular systems was good and therefore she did have a reasonable knowledge that could be built upon. Ellen started to feel less stupid and more in control of what she was doing. She could visualise herself as a nurse again and thoughts of quitting vanished. Ellen had also learned that her study technique needed adjusting. By focusing on the learning outcomes of the module, she could be more confident of achieving what was necessary to pass the exam. Ellen had learned a valuable lesson, namely how to deal with disappointment and still keep going. She became more resilient to adversity as a result.

This case study demonstrates that transitional space is a place where we learn and develop, sometimes in painful ways, by how we deal with different situations, and also that, as a result, we become changed as people. It is through constantly reviewing the interaction between our subjective experience and the feedback from the external world that we are able to develop. The external world relates to the people we interact with and the circumstances we have to deal with. By undertaking Activity 5.1 you will be able to identify where transitional space might be located within your own life and how you are learning and changing as a person.

Activity 5.1   Reflection

Try to remember a time of significant change or learning in your life and answer the following questions.

- What were the circumstances?
- How did you feel at the time?
- What did you learn?
- What change was brought about?
- Have you changed as a person as a result of the event?
- How did what you learned influence the change?
- Have you noticed any further changes and when and where have these occurred?

There is an outline answer to this activity at the end of the chapter.

This activity is likely to have focused on personal circumstances, on how you have developed as a person before and during your nurse preparation programme (and subsequent to it if you are an experienced practitioner), and on learning. Learning in different ways from those you are used to is itself a transitional space, as you are challenged to adjust your subjective meaning of what is being asked. Having identified where transitional spaces have appeared in your own life, we now proceed to consider what might be some of the barriers and limitations to being able to reflect and learn in such spaces.

Barriers and limitations to reflection

While reflection offers an opportunity for students and experienced practitioners to develop their own learning, nevertheless it may become inhibited by certain challenges. Some of the difficulties that may create barriers to reflection include:

- not knowing how to reflect – you get stuck with how things feel and cannot make sense of things;
- tiredness – too much effort is required to maintain mental focus;
- lack of time – life gets in the way;
- lack of insight – it is difficult to recognise how personal actions might affect others;
- distractions – it is difficult to find a quiet space;
- lack of motivation – you cannot see the relevance of reflection;
- finding it difficult to deal with the consequences of reflection – reflection is too painful or revealing.

Even when you are able to engage in reflection, there may be factors that lead to limitations in the reflection achieved. According to Smith and Jack (2005), these constitute the following.

- Learning styles – some learning styles are likely to help to engage with reflection in more meaningful ways than others.
- It is not easy for practitioners to articulate the knowledge they have – you may not be able to discern the decision-making thoughts of your supervisors.
- Reflection may be used for instrumental purposes and discontinued – reflection may remain focused on a course requirement.

Some of these aspects relate to personal knowledge of what reflection is about and what your role is within the process. Such barriers can be remedied by deepening your knowledge of reflection through reading. Other issues, such as having the time and space for reflection, can be overcome through organisation and negotiation. This in itself takes effort and motivation, which may come from realising that this is an opportunity to design your own learning. Limitations to reflection are likely to relate to the depth of reflection achieved. When reflection is a superficial process, which, perhaps, follows a reflection cycle without really analysing what is happening and why, then it remains limited.

Another way of overcoming some of the barriers and limitations to reflection is to ask your mentor to help you with reflective processing. This means being able to share your thinking and meaning making with your supervisor in a way that debates and discusses your thinking as something that is developing. This can be exposing in what it reveals of your 'becoming' to others, but is an important part of demonstrating progression and articulating how you are applying your knowledge in different situations. Consideration of how you might do this in diverse healthcare settings now follows.

Negotiating your place in diverse healthcare settings

A key aspect of 'becoming' is by negotiating your position in diverse healthcare settings. This takes place through developing your role and idea of who you need to be in different arenas. For example, the role of the nurse in an accident and emergency (A & E) department will be very different from that of a nurse working in the community setting. In A & E, the nurse's role is focused on problem solving (usually as quickly as possible). In the person's own home the nurse will be working collaboratively with the patient and this may take longer. While you are likely to be caring and empathic in both situations, you may nevertheless also need to be more assertive in A & E, which will bring about a different development. Part of the process of negotiating your position is to understand your role relevant to your stage of preparation within the particular setting. This involves:

- preparing for entering into the new setting – identifying key care priorities of the setting and getting to know the potential learning opportunities;
- reflecting on your current knowledge – mapping your knowledge to that of the care priorities of the setting and planning to address any deficits, possibly through drafting a **learning contract** if you are a student;
- reflecting on what you are doing, the feedback you are getting and how you might see yourself developing, while you are in the care setting;
- summarising what you have learned about the care setting and yourself, when moving on;
- reflecting on how any knowledge you have gained might be applicable in different settings you have experienced.

Preparation, reflecting and summarising are important features in helping to make sense of developing meaning from different settings. Undertaking Activity 5.2 will provide you with the opportunity to apply and think about some of these issues in relation to your own experiences, in order to develop learning from those experiences.

Activity 5.2   *Reflection*

Consider the different placements you have had (or if you are an experienced practitioner the different positions you have held). How did you:

- prepare for the placement or role;
- identify others' expectations of you;
- understand your position in the setting;
- develop your learning in the setting;
- develop your identity;
- feel when you left the setting and why did you feel that way;
- plan what to do next?

As this activity is based on your own experiences, there is no outline answer at the end of the chapter.

You may have identified that you left some settings with a more positive feeling than others. By working through how you prepared to enter the setting, reflecting on what you learned and your developing identity while you were there, you are able to connect the past with the present and a potential future. This is an important part of negotiating your position in a transitional space.

The second aspect of negotiating your position relates to the levels of dependence and independence that you may adopt, or be allowed to take on, in your working. When negotiating our position, previous experiences, as highlighted in Chapter 3, can influence our perceptions of others and ourselves (Winnicott, 1965). This may result in projecting the role of parent on to the supervisor, which can distort some of our responses. This process is illustrated within the following scenario.

Scenario: Ravi's experience of two mentors

Ravi was at the start of the third year of his nurse preparation programme and was working on a ward that specialised in diabetes. He had to return to this ward as he had to make up placement time he had lost due to sickness. While on this placement he was due to complete an assessment. His mentor, Sylvia, had been quite critical about his performance during his previous placement. Sylvia was again his mentor and Ravi felt very apprehensive as she had asked to have a formal meeting with him.

During their discussion, Sylvia commented that Ravi was still not meeting her expectations of his assessment objectives. She went through these in detail and identified that Ravi needed constant guidance. At this stage Sylvia was expecting that Ravi should be able to organise the care of a number of patients and hand over to others independently. She was concerned about whether Ravi was going to be able to pass the assessment and told him he needed to become more proactive in his dealings with patients and staff.

Ravi tried to explain that he knew what to do but wanted to confirm that this was correct. On leaving the meeting with Sylvia, Ravi felt demoralised and not sure what he could do to improve. He felt that everything he did was wrong. Ravi was due to work with another supervisor for the next two weeks as Sylvia was on leave.

Ravi met with his new mentor, Jane, on the Monday of the following week. Jane explained which patients she wanted Ravi to look after and organise the care for, and asked Ravi to tell her what he saw as the main priorities. Intermittently Jane would join Ravi for aspects of care such as the drug round, or when the consultant needed to see a patient, or during handover. She allowed Ravi to give the main information and would add points as necessary. By the end of the first week Ravi's confidence had grown. He began to think that he could pass this assessment as Jane told him he was working more independently. On the last week of his placement Sylvia was not available, so Jane undertook Ravi's assessment. Although there were a few areas in which she suggested he could develop further, Jane was satisfied that Ravi had passed his assessment.

Question

- In what ways were Ravi's responses distorted? What else could he have done to help in negotiating his position?

There is an outline answer to this question at the end of the chapter.

As is noted in this scenario, the quality of interactions can have a profound effect on our responses and ability to learn. When we are treated in negative ways we may also respond less confidently. Part of creating spaces for reflection includes using care and compassion when doing so in order to create a meaningful space for learning. We proceed now to consider issues relating to care and compassion within spaces of reflection.

Care and compassion

Care and compassion in terms of learning relate to how cared for you feel yourself to be. Nursing practice can sometimes be so hectic that you barely have time to think and feel under constant pressure. Creating space for reflection is a form of care that allows you to take stock of what is happening and grasp the opportunity to learn. Creating space for yourself to reflect is a form of self-caring that enables you to come to a different view of yourself (Schmidt, 2008). Equally, biographical construction and reflection, as discussed in Chapter 3, has the potential to change impressions and develop your learning in more affirming ways that are compassionate. The ability to explore the self is an important element of self-caring (Chan and Schwind, 2006). Undertaking Activity 5.3 might help you to read situations differently and see the opportunities for becoming self-caring.

Activity 5.3   *Critical thinking*

Look again at the case study of Ellen's failure (pages 68–9) and the above scenario of Ravi's experience of two mentors and consider the following.

*   Who showed care and compassion?
*   How were care and compassion demonstrated, if at all?
*   What were the results for Ellen and Ravi?
*   What did they take forward from their situations?
*   If care and compassion are absent, what is, or is likely to be, the outcome?
*   How can we show care and compassion for ourselves and others as part of reflection?

There are outline answers to this activity at the end of the chapter.

When you have completed answering the above points, write a reflective summary of what you have learned using the pro forma from Chapter 1 (page 18). Include an action plan for how you can show care and compassion.

As this activity is based on your learning experience, there is no outline answer at the end of the chapter.

Through undertaking the activity you are likely to have viewed the situations in more positive and affirmative ways. Reading situations from such a perspective can help to open up a space that is more compelling for learning, not in a coercive sense, but in being open-minded and engaged. We proceed now to consider such a space for reflection and learning, which draws all the parts already discussed into a whole.

Space that is compelling for reflection and learning

Space might be described as a ***compelling space*** (Horowitz, 2004, p155), where people initiate opportunities by engaging with one another to learn something new. Such acts of initiation might relate to you choosing whether or not to reflect, and so learn, and to the design that you give to your reflection. In other words, do you choose to reflect with others, in written form or by thinking things through on your own? A compelling space is one that invites meaningful learning and is where people feel able to acknowledge that they do not know (Howatson-Jones, 2010). In such a space you are empowered to become proactive in developing enquiry and meaning. It is here that real autonomy may be found in how you develop your own knowledge and take control of your learning. To do this you need to integrate the personal with the professional, as outlined in Chapter 3, and so create a compelling space. The following case study offers an example of how a compelling space is created.

Case study: Jared's experience of a compelling space

Jared was at the end of his nurse preparation programme and was working in an ambulatory cancer care centre. He really enjoyed this placement because there did not seem to be any hierarchical distinctions between the medical and nursing staff. They all worked as a team in a person-centred way. A poem written by one of the patients was displayed in the colourful waiting area and seemed to sum up these impressions in the prose used. Jared looked at this poem every day when he came on duty and it inspired him. Before finishing the placement his mentor, Abby, asked Jared to share his reflections and learning with the team. Inspired by the poem and the person-centred attitude of the team, Jared began with the poem that had so inspired him and his reflections emanating from this and his observations of the team and his learning about person-centredness. The team gave Jared positive feedback. He left the placement feeling affirmed and valued. When writing his reflective diary at home that night he considered what had helped his learning. It was a mix of the positive atmosphere, the team working together, the inspiration of the poem that had motivated him and the team's feedback on his practice. All these combined to make the space compelling for his learning.

Chapter summary

This chapter has introduced the concept of transitional space and offered you the opportunity to examine some transitional spaces in your own life through the activities provided. By exploring some of the barriers and limitations to reflection, suggestions for how to overcome these have also been illuminated and can be employed to help you increase your reflective opportunities. By examining how you negotiate your place within diverse healthcare settings, issues of care and compassion have been raised in how these influence the quality of the learning experience. By empowering individuals, compelling spaces for learning and reflection are created. The next chapter will continue this theme by looking at reflection and reflexivity.

Activities and scenarios: Brief outline answers

Activity 5.1: Reflection (page 69)

In considering the question about significant change in your life, you might have thought about when you were an adolescent, or maybe when you became a parent for the first time. Some of the feelings evoked are likely to have been anxiety and uncertainty. You might have learned new skills and this in turn may have helped you to grow in confidence. You are likely to have become increasingly independent and able to make decisions for yourself. Modifications to this change are likely to have ensued from problems you encountered and successes you experienced, so that there will have been further uncertain times, but also greater ability to direct your progression.

Activity 5.3: Critical thinking (page 73)

Your answers might have included the following.

- You might have identified that Mitch showed care and compassion towards Ellen in the case study, and Jane showed care and compassion in her working with Ravi in the scenario.
- Care and compassion were demonstrated by Mitch in helping Ellen to revise, and by Jane in supervising Ravi at key points in his work to ensure that he was not undermined but supported.
- Ellen was able to adjust her study and revision techniques, and Ravi was able to function in a more independent way.
- Ellen had become more resilient to adversity and Ravi was able to see himself as a capable practitioner.
- In the absence of care and compassion, people feel diminished and less capable and are more liable to make mistakes.
- Showing care and compassion for ourselves involves getting to know ourselves better through some of the techniques suggested in this book. Showing care and compassion for others involves looking for positives rather than being critical in negative ways.

Scenario: Brett's day with the community mental health nurse (page 67)

You might have considered the following activities as offering scope for reflection.

- Talking about practice with others – reflecting on observed practice and how this compared with knowledge.
- Talking about the day with others – highlighting positives and areas for further reflection.
- Working as part of a new team – reflecting on differences between settings.

The spaces that you might have identified as being potentially available for reflection include:

- while eating breakfast – current knowledge base being taken into the new setting;
- while cycling – what to find out about;
- between visits – what new knowledge has been gained;
- while exercising – revisiting new knowledge;
- when completing an assignment – how new knowledge might relate to the assignment.

You might not have taken up these opportunities for reflection because of a lack of time, or because you wanted to do something else, or because you were tired.

Scenario: Ravi's experience of two mentors (page 72)

Ravi's previous experience on the ward, working with Sylvia, had been anxiety provoking because of her constant criticism of him. Therefore he was adopting a child role of waiting to be told what to do in order to get things right. He perceived Sylvia in a parent role of knowing best. With Jane, Ravi was able to gradually move to a more grown-up role and perception that he could make decisions, but Jane was still available should he come across something he did not understand. Ravi could also have spoken to the university tutor about his experience as a way of helping him to negotiate his position.

Further reading

Honey, P and Mumford, A (2006) *The Learning Styles Questionnaire – 80 item version.* Maidenhead: Peter Honey.

This book explains different learning styles and offers the opportunity for identifying your own learning style.

Jarvis, P (2006) *Towards a Comprehensive Theory of Human Learning: Lifelong learning and the learning society, vol. 1.* London: Routledge.

This book offers a broad examination of different types of learning and is helpful for understanding how and why we learn.

Johns, C (2007) Deep in reflection. *Nursing Standard,* 21(38): 24–5.

This article explores the mutual benefits of reflecting with others.

Useful websites

www.bbc.co.uk/keyskills/extra/module1/1.shtml (BBC Key skills)

This website identifies different ways of learning relating to key skills.

www.open2.net/survey/learningstyles (BBC Learning styles)

This website offers another view of learning styles and includes an online survey to help you determine your style.

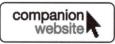

For further activities and other useful material, visit the companion website at **www.sagepub.co.uk/howatson-jones_reflective2e**

Chapter 6
Reflection and reflexivity

NMC Standards for Pre-registration Nursing Education

This chapter will address the following competency:

Domain 4: Leadership, management and team working

4. All nurses must be self-aware and recognise how their own values, principles and assumptions may affect their practice. They must maintain their own personal and professional development, learning from experience, through supervision, feedback, reflection and evaluation.

NMC Essential Skills Clusters

This chapter will address the following ESCs:

Cluster: Care, compassion and communication

6. People can trust the newly registered graduate nurse to engage therapeutically and actively listen to their needs and concerns, responding using skills that are helpful, providing information that is clear, accurate, meaningful and free from jargon.

By the first progression point:

3. Always seeks to confirm understanding.

By the second progression point:

6. Uses strategies to enhance communication and remove barriers to effective communication, minimising risk to people from lack of or poor communication.

Cluster: Organisational aspects of care

12. People can trust the newly registered graduate nurse to respond to their feedback and a wide range of other sources to learn, develop and improve services.

By the first progression point:

1. Responds appropriately to compliments and comments.

By the second progression point:

4. Takes feedback from colleagues, managers and other departments seriously and shares the messages and learning with other members of the team.

Chapter aims

After reading this chapter you will be able to:

- describe reflective conceptualisation at different stages of professional preparation;
- demonstrate how reflexivity may change your awareness in new ways;
- identify developing insight;
- relate to the experiences of others.

Example story

Neil was in the first year of his nurse preparation programme and working in a nursing home. He noticed that some of the team talked about other members of staff in not very nice ways. There was a lot of gossiping and sniping behind people's backs. This affected the atmosphere within the home and the communication between some team members. Neil felt uncomfortable at times when they tried to draw him into these conversations. On one occasion, however, he had joined in because the person concerned had, Neil felt, been quite 'off' with him.

Neil decided to reflect on the situation. He considered why some people were being singled out in this way. He thought about what he had learned in university about issues such as team working, cultural differences, being genuine and transactional analysis. The manager of the nursing home had only recently been appointed and was making a number of changes. It was clear that many of the staff were not happy with these. Neil wondered if they were projecting their anxieties on to each other and responding to these by attacking what they saw as anxiety-provoking. In the process, Neil thought that some people were moving away from adult-to-adult communication, and were hitting out in a more childish way.

Neil decided that, even if he could not change others' behaviour, he could at least modify his own and, maybe through this, influence situations. Neil decided to try to respond in positive ways to others in an effort to make conversations more affirming. Consequently, when staff tried to tell him about other staff in hostile ways, Neil responded by offering an alternative point of view. This often halted the progression of increasingly hostile dialogue. Neil assumed that he too was probably being talked about, but by fostering a more positive view himself he felt less intimidated and more able to influence his relationships. Neil started to gain confidence in what he came to see as his informal leadership skills.

Introduction

The example offered above illustrates how we are able to influence our own relationships with people and that, sometimes, by modifying our own behaviour, we may be able to influence that of others and the situations in which we find ourselves. As you begin to progress through your preparation programme, so you also start to develop resources and skills that enable you to direct and modify some of your experiences. Taking ownership of situations and what is being learned empowers you to consider alternatives and to make changes.

This chapter begins by defining what reflexivity is, and then proceeds to offer opportunities for you to examine how you can influence your experiences and how those experiences might influence you. The focus is on the role of reflexivity in developing opportunities for learning.

What is reflexivity?

Reflexivity can be defined as reflecting on the specifics of situations, as well as the conditions from which they arise, and how we might be implicated in those conditions. This requires you to examine the surrounding factors of how situations arise and in what ways your reflections might help you to influence your experiences, as well as how those experiences might shape you as a person and a practitioner. Reflexivity involves a continuous review of personal action to enact change (Alheit and Dausien, 2007). To do this requires you to examine your personal actions within the context of wider social interactions. For example, you are a developing practitioner within a wider profession, which has rules and regulations and expectations of its practitioners, but which also is represented by those practitioners. In this way it becomes possible for you to open up opportunities to consider how you are influencing your learning and how this is also influenced by life and social patterns. For example, how you study for exams will in part be influenced by the ways you have found successful in the past, but also by how your peer group perceives the concept of studying.

Equally, part of reflexivity is recognising that knowledge and knowing are integrated with the self. In other words, knowing is not separate from you as a person and what you bring to your understanding at a given time. For example, the culture you grew up in will have been influential in shaping who you are and how you perceive things, as discussed in Chapter 3. This is part of a **socialisation** process that continues throughout life (Jarvis, 2007). Culture and socialisation may influence your perceptions of what is similar to your view, of what is different and of what is classified as important. This will have become modified by other cultures such as school and working life. The professional culture and contexts of nursing will further alter your sense of self and how you integrate knowledge and knowing. Socialisation into the profession and its body of knowledge sets boundaries that start to become defended when working with others (Ousey and Johnson, 2007). Anxiety, fear and overemphasis on results can lead to focusing on a tick-box approach to the completion of learning tasks, but not on actually accomplishing learning. Reflexivity, as a consequence, can therefore become limited and superficial when other priorities take over. Reflexivity involves 'mindfulness', which means paying attention to situations, staff conduct and practice contexts to monitor for potential problems and solutions (Iedema, 2011).

Consider the following scenario to identify how reflexivity may become limited between teams.

Scenario: Sue's experience of fragmenting teams

Sue was in the second year of her nurse preparation programme and working on an orthopaedic ward. The ward next door was often short-staffed, and the qualified nurses from Sue's ward were frequently asked to cover. Staff on Sue's ward helped each other out by coming in earlier or going home later. They were resentful that the ward next door did not seem to do the same and that they had to help them. Sue observed that this started to affect relationships and cause tensions. The hostile atmosphere also affected opportunities to learn.

Sue observed that, on her ward, there were numerous opportunities for learning as the staff constantly shared practice and reflected on what they were doing. The ward manager had set up a programme of lunchtime sessions where they could do this, and this included other professionals who came in to talk about their perspectives as well. However, it was interesting that the staff did not appear to be reflecting on the relationship with the other ward and Sue started to think about why this might be.

It seemed that there were different cultures on the two different wards. On Sue's ward, the manager was very proactive in trying to support learning and her staff. On the other ward, staff felt that they had little say in their working life and seemed to experience less support. Sue came to this conclusion because one of her friends was working on the other ward. Sue wondered whether the perceived lack of support was why staff were reluctant to give up any more of their own time and whether this was contributing to the atmosphere between the wards.

Sue considered the difference in attitude between the wards in terms of being a nurse and what this meant to her. She had come into nursing because she saw helping people as a vocation rather than a job. To Sue, this meant that, if patients needed some extra time, it might require her staying behind beyond the end of a shift. Having been brought up to help people, Sue saw this as a normal part of her role. She felt she could understand the resentment of the staff on her ward, as she perceived the other ward staff were not contributing as much and sometimes took advantage as they knew they would get help.

Question

- Looking at this scenario reflexively, what other interpretations might you have? What area of commonality might offer the potential for the staff to forge a different relationship?

There is an outline answer to this question at the end of the chapter.

This scenario might have helped you to identify that, even when we are reflecting, we often do not think reflexively about situations, how culture influences us and what this contributes to the circumstances we encounter.

By undertaking Activity 6.1 you will be able to develop some insight into how culture influences your reflexive thinking.

Activity 6.1   *Critical thinking*

When thinking about the different cultures you have experienced at home, at school, through your friends and professionally, consider the following questions.

- How have the various cultures influenced you?
- What is important to you in learning to be a nurse?
- How does your background influence your views of learning as a nurse?
- What kind of knowledge is important to you and why do you think it is important?
- How do you develop knowing?
- How has developing as a nurse professional affected the kind of knowledge you see as important?

There is an outline answer to this activity at the end of the chapter.

Through completing the activity you may have identified some influences on the way you perceive things and what is important. In this way you are able to develop awareness of how your thinking is shaped and how you can start to exert some influence on modifying your thinking and circumstances. We proceed now to consider the process of taking ownership.

Taking ownership

Taking ownership means taking responsibility for your own action or inaction. In other words, in terms of reflection and reflexivity, this means being responsible for examining issues and being honest with yourself in what you contribute to the situation and what the outcomes say about your approach. By recognising your own participation it will become clearer where adjustments might be needed, or might make the most contribution. The process of taking ownership involves:

- developing self-awareness;
- communicating developmental needs;
- using emotional intelligence;
- becoming historically and politically aware;
- informing yourself.

Personal insight and self-awareness are the cornerstones of reflexivity (Lee, 2009). Self-awareness relates to being attuned to what makes up the inner world (van Ooijen, 2003); in other words, how you really think and feel about things and what values you might have. Superficial approaches to reflection and reflexivity are sometimes used as ways of avoiding ownership, as their instrumental purpose and limited analysis circumvent challenging the **self-concept**, and also, therefore, do not result in any lasting change. The experienced practitioner who has developed personal insight and self-awareness will nevertheless remain alert to the reactions of others to their interventions in order to continue learning. Communication is the key to ensuring that perceptions are accurate, and to exploring the best way to move forward.

Communicating your developmental needs to others is part of the skills set you need to build up during your preparation programme. Nursing practitioners are expected to be self-aware about their knowledge and competence, and to address any deficits (NMC, 2008). It is through reflection that such deficits will come to light in meaningful ways for you, even if they were highlighted by others, such as your mentor. You will have learned communication skills as part of your nurse preparation programme, by looking at basic theories in the first year and how to apply these in different settings throughout the rest of the programme. Nursing communication needs to be both therapeutic and professional in relation to how you communicate with patients and other professionals when organising care (Sully and Dallas, 2005). However, communicating your needs is a part of this and might be difficult when you lack confidence, or have concerns about how you are perceived by others. Even experienced practitioners might fear acknowledging developmental needs. Taking ownership of your needs is an important aspect of being a nursing practitioner and requires:

- seeking appropriate support and guidance;
- dealing with your emotions constructively;
- addressing knowledge gaps;
- undertaking independent study.

Nursing involves emotional labour because it deals with people who live emotional lives. Emotional intelligence is having awareness of one's own emotions and being able to read the emotional cues of others (Spinks, 2009). When first starting your nursing preparation programme you may have been aware of your own emotional reactions, but were possibly less proficient in reading those of others. As you develop through the programme you will find yourself 'tuning in' to the emotional states of your clients and patients. In a similar way, these skills can be brought to reading situations reflectively by 'tuning in' to the emotional vibrations that resonate through the situation and the language that you and others use to describe it. Using emotional intelligence means being able to distinguish stressors and work that is emotionally meaningful and how internal values are aligned with these (Price, 2008). The early portion of your reflection will almost certainly be aroused by emotion, but unless emotional intelligence is activated to read the situation and people's reactions, reflection will remain mired in feelings and not move forward to actual learning. Part of such attunement requires being aware of what has gone before in order to be alert to cues in the present.

Historical insight is an important part of this process. For example, if you are aware that a particular unit has undergone considerable change in previous years, it will not surprise you to find that some staff may be resistant to further alterations. Equally, political changes have a profound effect on healthcare priorities and resources, and these are equally influential in how supported, or not, practitioners feel themselves to be. It is sometimes easy within reflection to make assumptions about situations and their solutions without a historical and political perspective, and where reflective solutions in reality are unworkable and therefore lead to further frustration. Part of guarding against this circumstance is to inform yourself of the background and context of the situation and some of the surrounding issues, and to ensure that your knowledge pertaining to these is up to date. Informing yourself may require some independent study and consequently time, which will need to be factored into your learning plan. Consider the following scenario to identify processes of taking ownership of reflection and reflexivity.

Scenario: Geeta's experience of developing ownership in reflection

Geeta was in the final year of her nurse preparation programme and working in an operating theatre environment. She was on her last extended placement and was hoping to secure a permanent post as a theatre nurse practitioner after qualifying. Geeta had been in this placement for five weeks when a second-year student, Joe, was also placed there for a shorter time, as part of his acute care experience. Geeta did not really get on with Joe as she found him rather patronising, and it appeared that some of the other staff also did not like him very much. Geeta's mentor asked her to help orientate Joe to the theatre suite and the ways of working, as she felt that Joe might respond more positively to another student.

Geeta found that Joe acted as if he was in charge as he tried to take over things that Geeta normally did. The patients seemed to like Joe, though, as he had a good patient manner that put them at ease when they arrived looking nervous. Joe tended to want to be in the thick of the most complicated cases and this sometimes limited Geeta's opportunities.

On this particular day Geeta and Joe were working in the same theatre. Geeta had helped to set up the instrument trolley with her mentor, and both she and Joe were now helping to set up the staff with their final requirements. The operation commenced and Geeta and Joe were invited to view the surgeon's actions more closely. On turning round, Geeta noticed that Joe had accidentally touched part of the instrument trolley and potentially desterilised it. Geeta had no option but to tell the scrub nurse, which she attempted to do as discreetly as possible. However, the trolley needed to be changed and this caused a short delay and was noticeable to everyone.

After the operation was completed, Geeta was helping to clean up in the dirty area. When Geeta was alone, Joe came in and angrily told Geeta she had made him look really stupid and how dare she show him up. Geeta explained why it had been necessary to change the trolley. Joe replied that it was not up to her and she was getting above her place. At this point, feeling under attack, Geeta told Joe that she found his attitude difficult at times, a view shared by some of the staff. Joe grabbed a passing qualified nurse and asked her if this was true. The nurse replied that there were times when he appeared not to listen to people. Joe stormed out of the room.

Geeta had to take a short break as she felt very upset by this incident. On her way home that evening she started to reflect on the experience. Geeta was confident that she had taken the right action, but was less sure about telling Joe that other staff found him difficult. She also wondered whether part of her reaction was due to her own difficulties with him.

Question

- If you were Geeta, how and where would you start to take ownership of this reflection? What particular elements of the scenario would you draw on as being particularly important?

There is an outline answer to this question at the end of the chapter.

This scenario might have helped you to think about your reflections using emotional intelligence to better discern the perspectives of others. Reflexivity means that we are able to judge the effects of our actions on others as much as the effects they may have on us. We proceed now to consider the role of reflexivity in developing learning.

Role of reflexivity in developing learning

The role of reflexivity in learning has been defined as how students or nurse practitioners orientate themselves to learning opportunities (Cassidy, 2009). Such orientation involves bringing personal knowledge to the caring situation, at the same time as recognising what meaning is made from the situation and related knowledge. To do this requires:

- being aware of internal dialogue;
- embedding learning through integration;
- recognising the relatedness of knowledge;
- having awareness of nursing as a community of practice.

To be aware of an internal dialogue means listening to internal reasoning processes, meaning and decision making. For example, you might be involved in an assessment discussion with your mentor in which you are talking about how you communicate with patients. Your mentor may highlight particular techniques that need to be used, but that you know how to use. You might identify that your meaning and your mentor's interpretation of these techniques is at variance and that you need to decide how to proceed. Throughout the conversation you will be aware of a running internal commentary. Some call this commentary an internal mentor (Percival, 2001) and this internal dialogue may either help or hinder the outcome of your deliberations, depending on how in harmony it is with, or how divergent it is from, your thinking and acting. This process is a part of integrating learning.

Integrating learning means drawing together different strands of knowing and knowledge gained through the complex business of nursing (Zander, 2007). The integration process involves reflection, including listening for the internal commentary as explained above, in order to embed new information and connect it to that already in place. The connections are made through reflecting on what is brought to situations, what is taken away from them and how well things went. This is part of the process of integrating learning previously explained in Chapter 3. Imagining connects here to the internal dialogue that assesses possible consequences of actions. In this way knowledge starts to be related rather than simply accumulated.

Relating knowledge also makes it easier to apply it to different situations. For example, relating knowledge of different communication techniques makes it possible to understand how some might, for instance, be more applicable to a short-term setting than others. Equally, relating knowledge of physiological effects of virus invasion on the body with knowledge of economic and social pressures makes it easier to understand contrary behaviours and the prolonging of infection. Understanding the evolvement of theories and concepts helps to develop a reflexive frame by which these may also be questioned. Theories are suppositions that develop learning when questioned through reflexive thinking. Without such questioning, theories remain dormant in terms of learning and, consequently, are not easily recalled or applied. Part of being a reflexive practitioner is to help develop theories through different applications within the community of nursing.

Nursing is part of a community of practice through sharing a common purpose of caring for people. People exist within a *community of practice* (Wenger, 1998, p6) in the way they organise themselves and their lives. Nursing, as a community, offers the possibility for integrating practice with academic knowledge through providing engagement that questions both theory and practice (Andrew et al., 2008). As a developing nurse practitioner you are embedding learning in that community of practice through the ideas you reciprocally work through your university programme and practice. The capacity to be reflexive within your community determines how successful this process is. Collaborating reflexively within a community of practice helps you as a student, and the supervising practitioner, to learn both personally and as professionals. Sharing ideas in a community of practice helps them to develop and ensures practice is dynamic rather than stagnating.

Consider the following scenario to identify processes of reflexive development of learning.

Scenario: Ashley's reflexive learning experience

Ashley was in the first year of his nurse preparation programme and was working with the community nurses for his third placement. He had learned clinical observation skills and how to complete a simple assessment in the hospital environment, but was unsure how these translated to the community setting. Ashley voiced this concern with his mentor, Miranda, on his first day. Miranda reassured Ashley that for the first week she would be expecting him to observe her and complete simple nursing observations while he was orientating himself to the community environment. Ashley observed how Miranda always had a laugh with the patients and the easy therapeutic relationship she established with them. He also observed how clear her explanations were for the patients and also for him when he asked her about the use of different tools and told her what he had been taught.

At the end of the first week Ashley and Miranda reflected on the week's learning for both of them. Ashley told Miranda what he had observed about her communication style. Miranda in turn highlighted how valuable she found Ashley's presence for making her think about the explanation for what she was doing and helping her to develop her teaching practice through sharing his learning and knowledge. Ashley was surprised by this as Miranda seemed so knowledgeable to him. Her last statement that there was always something to learn made him think.

Question
• What reflexive learning is taking place here for Ashley and Miranda?

There is an outline answer to this question at the end of the chapter.

Chapter summary

This chapter has begun to define reflexivity. By offering activities that ask the novice and developing nurse to consider how they employ reflexivity, the chapter has offered opportunities to make sense of internal dialogue and cultural considerations within the wider community of nursing. Through inclusion of examples of how to take ownership of reflective and reflexive processes and what they may reveal, the chapter has made it possible

continued . . .

to develop real insight, and increase self-awareness and consequently the effectiveness of the practitioner. By underpinning this with developing emotional intelligence you have the possibility for reading situations more reflexively and integrating this knowledge differently to develop caring. The importance of this as a part of reflective practice will be continued in the next chapter.

Activities and scenarios: Brief outline answers

Activity 6.1: Critical thinking (page 81)

When completing the activity you might have highlighted some of the following points.

- Home and school are likely to have influenced your approach to studying and learning in more or less positive ways.
- Learning the skills of being a nurse is likely to be a priority for you.
- Your background may have given you a view of learning as a nurse that differs concerning practical and academic contributions.
- Practical knowledge may be of greater importance than academic knowledge, or scientific knowledge may be a greater priority than softer skills such as communication, because this is the evidence base for your actions.
- Your knowing is likely to develop by doing, as well as through sharing your practice and reflecting.
- Developing as a nurse professional is likely to have identified the importance of a variety of knowledge, spanning the psychological, sociological, biological, ethical, spiritual, personal and professional.

Scenario: Sue's experience of fragmenting teams (page 80)

While Sue's background had laid the foundation for helping her to view nursing as a vocation, life circumstances for some people might also get in the way. Equally, nursing is a highly skilled profession that deserves to be remunerated. Both sets of staff appeared to feel coerced into working in a different way, provoking anxiety and making it more difficult for them to think reflexively. When thinking reflexively, Sue might see that, if the situation of helping out the ward next door continued indefinitely, they might never get the resources they needed in terms of extra staff. Perhaps this could offer a starting point for dialogue between the two wards, in how they might address this in the longer term together and so develop a more positive relationship. Talking in this way might also help them to share practice and through this develop learning opportunities.

Scenario: Geeta's experience of developing ownership in reflection (page 83)

In the scenario, Geeta is aware of her own responsibilities and those of Joe in terms of maintaining sterility. She clearly understands the processes, but Joe appears to be less certain. The first aspect for Geeta to reflect on is the relationship between her and Joe, and between Joe and the other staff. It might have been useful at the first signs of problems to have discussed with Joe how he had got on in other placements, to see if there was some reason for his attitude. Geeta needs also to consider their differing developmental needs and whether these have been adequately discussed with their mentors, as it appears that their needs are being amalgamated and this is limiting Geeta's learning.

The main portion of Geeta's reflection needs to consider her limited use of emotional intelligence. She is aware of her own emotional reactions, but not those of others. How was Joe feeling when he entered the theatre environment and might his behaviour have been bravado? Were Joe's feelings administered to directly after the incident? Geeta needed to review how she could have taken responsibility for being concerned with her own feelings more than Joe's. She might have acknowledged that she felt her position of trust by the theatre staff was threatened by Joe, and led to her reaction of telling Joe about the negative views of some staff, thus escalating the situation. Geeta might need to read about exercising emotional intelligence to inform her practice.

Scenario: Ashley's reflexive learning experience (page 85)

Ashley's presence helped Miranda to focus on the quality of her explanation for the benefit of Ashley and the patient. She was also re-examining her knowledge base in the light of Ashley's questions. Ashley was reviewing his present knowledge to identify what adjustments he needed to make for applying it in this new care context. He was influenced by Miranda's communication style, which he viewed as a positive role model for practice.

Further reading

Cassidy, S (2009) Interpretation of competence in student assessment. *Nursing Standard*, 23(18): 39–46.

This article will help you to understand how mentors use reflexivity in coming to assessment decisions and how important reflexivity is in developing competence as a nurse.

Goleman, D (2004) *Emotional Intelligence & Working with Emotional Intelligence* (omnibus). London: Bloomsbury.

This book will help you to understand the relationship between emotions and cognition and the importance of working with emotional intelligence when dealing with people.

Sully, P and Dallas, J (2005) *Essential Communication Skills for Nursing*. Edinburgh: Elsevier Mosby.

This book helps to identify how you can develop appropriate communication skills for therapeutic and professional purposes.

Reflective Practice (**journal**)

This journal offers a variety of articles on difference aspects of reflecting and practising reflexively.

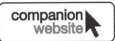

For further activities and other useful material, visit the companion website at **www.sagepub.co.uk/howatson-jones_reflective2e**

Chapter 7
The reflective practitioner

continued . . .

Cluster: Organisational aspects of care

11. People can trust the newly registered graduate nurse to safeguard children and adults from vulnerable situations and support and protect them from harm.

By the first progression point:

2. Shares information with colleagues and seeks advice from appropriate sources where there is a concern or uncertainty.

Chapter aims

After reading this chapter you will be able to:

* define and identify morally active practice;
* recognise the fallibility of professional knowledge and developing practice;
* develop some strategies to manage knowledge deficits, near misses and mistakes in your practice;
* understand the need for reflecting on the complexity of decisions and consequences.

Example story

Debbie was in the third year of her nurse preparation programme. She was on a specialist placement with the **multiple sclerosis** (MS) nurse, Gill. Debbie was very interested in seeing how Gill worked with a caseload of her own patients, referring them to other health professionals as appropriate. This was a different view of nursing and one Debbie was not familiar with. She thought about what she had observed from seeing Gill working with a variety of patients with differing degrees of illness severity. Debbie was surprised that, at times, Gill acknowledged to patients that she was not sure what was causing their symptoms, but that working together they would be able to devise an appropriate plan. When Debbie had asked about this, Gill had highlighted that patients were the experts in terms of what they were experiencing and their coping strategies. MS is such a variable illness and more is being discovered about it all the time.

Gill related the example of **benign MS**, which had been assumed not to cause significant nerve damage, and therefore patients developed milder symptoms that were usually non-progressive, and were often not taken seriously. However, recent research findings had suggested that far more significant damage was sustained within the first attack and could lie dormant until further illness and ageing activated damaged areas and potentially triggered progression. Gill used this example to explain to Debbie how important it was for the health practitioner to work with patients and constantly review their own assumptions of what was happening and what they were noticing. She also explained how it was most important to reflect on what they were doing and the aesthetics present within their practice.

Debbie realised that what she was experiencing was a reflective practitioner in action who was not afraid to acknowledge uncertainty, but who embraced it by reflecting with patients in a skilful way that drew out what was most concerning them and imaginatively working with possibilities. Supporting this was Gill's up-to-date knowledge base, caring and concern for her patients, and her ability to interpret and review complex issues. Debbie realised Gill was the type of role model practitioner she aspired to emulate.

Introduction

The example above demonstrates the changing nature of knowledge, and why it is important to reflect on practice in order to be able to respond effectively to change. The openness to work with change in practice is a fundamental feature of the reflective practitioner. If we accept that professionals are fallible and do not always get things right, we have a point from which to start to examine the effectiveness of practice by reflecting on what might be done differently. Equally, as clients are unique human beings they may not always respond in expected ways. Nevertheless, being open to change and reflecting on it allows the practitioner to learn and develop. It is important for students to be able to acknowledge limitations within their knowledge as well as to take ownership of potential mistakes through reflection, in order to learn how to be accountable and reflective practitioners.

This chapter links with another book in the series, *Evidence-based Practice in Nursing* (Ellis, 2013), and will encourage the student to cultivate a reflective approach to their daily experience, and integrate what they are learning with their practice. We begin by examining what morally active practice is.

Morally active practice

Morally active practice is defined as critically exercising decisions based on ethical and moral principles and being able to justify these (Brechin, 2000). The morally active practitioner recognises that there are situations when some influences, such as evidence and policy, may take precedence over others, such as personal values and patient preference, which might not be reasonable. However, some ethical principles (such as equity) must be applied, so the practitioner needs to be aware of the consequences of their actions (Ellis and Howatson-Jones, 2008). Our moral thinking is influenced by the cultures we have experienced and our own histories. Moral practice is informed by professional expectation and acceptability and concern for human beings with regard to the individual in that situation at that time.

It is important to be clear about our motives and the expected consequences of our actions, as well as being respectful about people's concerns and well-being. For example, you might have strong views about people smoking when they know it is harmful. This might translate into differing attitudes towards those presenting for treatment. Even if this is repressed, it may nevertheless still be active within your thinking and, therefore, reflecting. A more extreme example might be when faced with caring for someone who is an abuser, or a person who has inflicted some harm on themselves or others. Equity means that care should be provided immaterial of personal feelings or prejudices. However, reflecting on reactions to such situations is an important part of being able to deal with them, and of learning from the experience.

The morally active practitioner utilises a reflective rather than a judgemental approach to examine the outcomes of their actions and decisions. This is important when reflecting on actions that give rise to such hesitancy and for bringing everything into view. This also means using your whole self when thinking about practice, engaging feelings and being aware of intentions.

Activity 7.1   *Reflection*

Use the following questions to spend a little time reflecting on your own values and beliefs.

- What is important to you and why?
- What do you find difficult to bear and why?
- Have the answers to the above questions changed during the course of your life and, if so, why?
- How have these issues related to your practice?

There is an outline answer to this activity at the end of the chapter.

Professional experience is helpful for providing the skills necessary to develop, but it is also important to consider what we think about being a professional and how we interpret professionalism. For example, the fact that practitioners are able to negotiate freely the nursing environment, while patients and clients are not, puts you, as the practitioner, in a position of power. This needs to be considered with regard to how you approach your practice. Employing an authoritarian approach that places you firmly in control means that you may be cut off from learning other points of view, namely the patient's or others', which also inform practice and are useful for reflecting on. Equally, when you are just following instructions and policies you may appear to be professional, but if you omit reflection on your practice all you are doing is conforming to established behaviours. This is not the same as reflecting to ensure the effectiveness and development of practice. The following scenario will help to illustrate this point.

Scenario: Pavlina's professional experience

Pavlina was in the second year of her nurse preparation programme working in a radiology department. Everything was new to her and she was worried about the radiation involved in imaging procedures. Her mentor, Gabriel, asked her to read the radiation protection guidelines in her first week. Pavlina reflected after continued . . . •••

reading these. She thought about how she had felt on her first day and wondered whether patients might have similar feelings and concerns about radiation. She considered the new knowledge she had gained from reading the radiation protection guidelines and how these could inform her practice.

Pavlina observed a variety of diagnostic and interventional procedures, always making sure she was in position to reassure the patient. As the placement continued, she felt more confident to inform patients about what was happening. Gabriel involved her in setting up procedures and undertaking nursing observations. Pavlina learnt a lot during patient handovers to ward staff after interventional procedures as well. She was, however, concerned that these handovers took place in a public space.

Pavlina reflected with Gabriel at the end of her placement. Gabriel told her how impressed he was with the way that she had translated her reading of the radiation protection guidelines into reassuring explanations for the patients. He also praised Pavlina's hard work and dedication to her learning. Pavlina told Gabriel how much she had enjoyed the variety of learning opportunities available in this placement, but she also voiced concern about patient handovers occurring in public spaces and the way that the radiologists explained the procedure in the room and then asked the patient for their consent. Pavlina felt that this could be perceived as coercive as everyone was ready for the procedure to start. Gabriel reflected with Pavlina on these issues.

Questions

- What do you think Pavlina has learned about professionalism in this scenario?
- What else might she have learned about effective practice through reflection with Gabriel?
- What options for change might they have considered?

There are outline answers to these questions at the end of the chapter.

When reading the scenario above you may have immediately had some further questions and thoughts about what was happening. It is for this reason that Abrandt Dahlgren et al. (2004, p15) urge that practitioners reflect 'about' practice as well as 'on' or 'in' practice. By this they mean that practical awareness can only develop when such reflective thinking occurs and helps nursing as a profession to move forward. Taking responsibility for your own learning through reflecting about the practice you are involved in is an important part of this process. We proceed now to examine how professionals might sometimes be fallible and the role of reflection in managing this situation.

Practitioner fallibility and reflection

As a healthcare practitioner you are subjected to scrutiny from a number of directions. The NMC sets the standards for practice and regulates professional behaviour (NMC, 2008). The government legislates the policies with which healthcare is expected to comply (Department of Health (DH), 2009), and the Quality Assurance Agency (QAA, 2008) inspects the validity of teaching and assessment. With so many dictates for practice, it is hardly surprising that professionals sometimes get things wrong. Human error theory asserts that error is inevitable at some stage, but it is important to establish the reasons for flaws in judgement in order to address any problems (Armitage, 2009). Undertaking Activity 7.2 might help you to identify some issues that may play a part in potential practitioner fallibility and, with this knowledge, to reflect on how you might avoid these issues.

Activity 7.2 — *Critical thinking*

Think of a decision you made that you considered was a bad decision. Try to think of what might have interfered with your ability to make judgements and decisions by considering the following questions.

- What were the circumstances?
- What was the result?
- What do you think contributed to it being a bad decision?
- What did you do afterwards?
- What do you think about it now?

Using your previous answers, now consider how to make good decisions.

As this activity is based on your own experiences there are limited answers at the end of the chapter.

The decisions that professionals make usually require them to process information and use some level of intuition and cognitive aspects (Muir, 2004). Information processing refers to making sense of all the information available in terms of what is observed, heard, felt, smelt and read. Intuition refers to knowledge from experience being activated by the situation and inducing a response. Cognitive aspects relate to thinking about all of this and coming to a decision. During the process of deciding, choices are analysed in terms of their possible consequences, although sometimes we might not be wholly aware of this.

Social judgement theory suggests that the problem and informational cues link to the situation on which judgements are based. The ordering of importance of the cues determines how accurate the judgement is for the actual situation (Thompson and Dowding, 2002). Creativity through remaining flexible and responsive, using information-processing skills to understand emerging data, being clear about what you are aiming for, seeking guidance as appropriate, and knowing the extent and limits of your knowledge are all contributing factors to good decision making (Bohinc and Gradisar, 2003). By reading the following scenario and answering the question at the end you may be able to identify some issues relating to practitioner fallibility.

Scenario: Elsie's escapade

Rose was in the first year of her nurse preparation programme and working on a ward caring for older people. One of the patients, Elsie, was quite confused. On this particular day, Elsie was found to be missing from the ward and Rose joined her mentor, Mary, in searching for her. Elsie was eventually found down by continued . . .

the main road sitting on the grass. Rose and Mary collected Elsie, putting her in a wheelchair and returning her to the ward. As Elsie was cold, Rose helped her into bed to warm up. Mary asked Rose to complete a set of observations of Elsie's temperature, pulse and blood pressure to check on her and for entering into the clinical incident form. Rose recorded these and noted that Elsie's temperature was a little low, but nothing else appeared abnormal. The doctor was also informed of Elsie's escapade, but as she appeared not to have suffered any effects he told Mary to just continue to keep an eye on her. The rest of the day was uneventful, although Elsie was restless and would call out every so often. She eventually went to sleep that night.

Rose was on the early shift the next morning. As soon as she came on duty she heard Elsie wailing and crying. When she asked Mary what the problem was, Mary told her that Elsie had woken up in pain, and when the staff pulled her covers back they noticed that her left leg was externally rotated and shortened, a classic symptom of a fractured neck of femur. As Elsie had not been out of bed overnight (she had a urinary catheter) no one had noticed this deformity until Elsie woke in pain. Rose asked Mary how it was possible that they had missed this.

Elderly bones are more fragile than younger ones because mineral density decreases with age, so even a relatively minor fall can lead to a fracture. Sometimes the muscles that encircle the hip go into rigid spasm and this can, temporarily, hold the hip in reasonable alignment. When the body relaxes, as happens in sleep, the muscles no longer maintain their hold and the deformity becomes apparent. It is unlikely that Elsie would have been able to walk on this leg, but as she returned to the ward by wheelchair this also was not obvious.

Questions
- What contributed to practitioner fallibility in this scenario?
- What should or could have been done differently?
- What might be learned from this situation?

There are outline answers to these questions at the end of the chapter.

While the registered practitioner is accountable for their actions and those they are supervising, nevertheless the student is responsible for ensuring that they notify changes or deficits that they have become aware of. Reflection itself may be fallible when based on inaccurate perceptions. Schön (1987) makes the point that, when understanding is not grounded in proper practice through careful examination and checking of knowing, inaccurate ideas about practice may perpetuate because the reflection itself is flawed. Reflecting with others, as will be discussed in Chapter 8, and analytical approaches, such as those explored in Chapter 11, can help to combat such fallibility. We proceed now to consider how to manage near misses and mistakes.

Managing deficits and near misses or mistakes

Fragmented inter-nurse and interprofessional relations can make managing deficits difficult and lead to lack of communication between groups, creating working processes conducive to errors.

Equally, anxiety can hold back progress as a person finds it difficult to make a decision for fear of getting it wrong and therefore relies on being told what to do by others. Without the confidence and knowledge to interrogate your practice, and that of others, poor practice and mistakes may be perpetuated. The following case study helps to illustrate this point.

Rhian's experience of poor practice

Rhian was in the first year of her nurse preparation programme and on placement in a nursing home. She was keen to make a good impression and was anxious to do things correctly. A number of the patients had continence problems but, during the day, through careful observation and trips to the toilet, the problem was dealt with in a dignified way. But Rhian had started to notice, when she was on an early shift, that some of these patients had many incontinence pads in their beds, and that these were making their skin sweat and were consequently sticking to them. When Rhian mentioned this to a care assistant, the care assistant told her not to interfere as this was the way things were done on the night shift. Rhian was not sure about this, but did not want to make a fuss and show herself up. She decided to talk to her mentor about it. When Rhian spoke to her mentor, Dave, he said that it was different at night because the patients could not get up as easily to go to the toilet and so the pads were necessary. Rhian relayed that there seemed to be rather a lot of them and they were always very wet. Dave said he would look into it. However, the weeks passed and Rhian did not see any change. She was anxious that perhaps she had been wrong to think that this was not right. Rhian left her placement with the view that using a lot of incontinence pads at night was normal practice. Three months later, when reflecting after another placement, she realised that what she had seen in the first placement was wrong. She decided that if she was concerned about practice again she would challenge the practice and talk to her mentor, but she would also follow it up with a link tutor.

The case study has illustrated that, without reflection, practice and developing knowledge can be difficult. Developing reflective ability is a transitional process that involves struggle, accepting the challenge, making connections, learning to reflect more deeply and sharing with others (Glaze, 2001). Rhian could have progressed from her struggle with understanding, to accepting the challenge to find out more herself. This might, in turn, have helped her to make different connections and learn.

Mistakes can be a form of 'shocking' learning through their abrupt nature, which also triggers an emotional response. Mistakes can leave you feeling emotionally upset and can lower your self-esteem, unless this can be resolved and transformed into learning through reflection, supporting the regaining of self-confidence. This involves considering how action, or inaction, contributed to the error, thinking about the nature of the mistake and what it means to be a professional. Responses can be categorised as emotional, cognitive and behavioural as follows.

Emotional response

Stage 1   shock and grief;
Stage 2   defending by projecting blame.

Cognitive response

Stage 3   scrutinising own practice, acknowledging shortcomings;
Stage 4   scrutinising others' contributing practice to identify influences;
Stage 5   identifying the core problem and accepting responsibility;
Stage 6   checking core knowledge.

Behavioural response

Stage 7   reflecting on the error and behaviour and how to change;
Stage 8   identifying how to improve and regaining confidence.

It is important that emotional responses to difficult practice and errors are acknowledged at the start in order to be able to move forward to thinking about what needs to change. Consider the following scenario to think about how such transitional processes might occur.

Scenario: Roger's near miss

Roger was in the final year of his nurse preparation programme working on a day surgery unit. The pace of work at the start of the day was quite fast with many people arriving and needing to be prepared for theatre. Often premedications were required and had to be given quickly. One of the patients had been ready for a little while and Roger and his mentor, Sarah, went to get his premedication. They checked that it was prescribed and properly signed for by the doctor, that it had not already been given and that the patient had no allergies to the drug. They then checked the patient's name band and told him that the tablets they were giving him were his premedication. The patient's wife said that he had just been given tablets in the last ten minutes. When Sarah checked with the other staff she discovered that the patient had been given his premed previously, but that the nurse had forgotten to sign for it because she was busy. Due to the alertness of the patient's wife this had been a near miss. Sarah and Roger completed a critical incident form for this episode. Sarah reported the incident to the unit manager.

During a lull later in the morning Sarah and Roger reflected on this incident. Both of them felt quite shocked at the near miss and angry with the nurse who had not signed after giving the premedication. Roger discussed the merits of, in future, asking patients whether they had been given the premedication already, but Sarah pointed out that patients may not know what type of drugs they had already been given. Sarah highlighted that all professionals are fallible and that the only guard against this was to follow drug administration guidelines and to learn from such incidents. What they had both learned was to ensure that documentation was completed in a timely manner and to delegate tasks that might prevent this. Subsequent to this event Roger was very careful when checking any medication and also with his documentation.

Questions

- What learning did Roger take from this incident?
- In what ways are emotional, cognitive and behavioural responses evident in Sarah's and Roger's reflections?
- If you are an experienced practitioner how might the unit manager have dealt with this incident and the nurses involved?

There are outline answers to these questions at the end of the chapter.

Regaining confidence after a mistake requires support as well as guidance in order to be ready to identify where the point of departure from effective decision making comes. We proceed now to consider reflecting on complex decisions in order to assist with the process of identifying effectiveness.

Reflecting on complex decisions

Practice experiences incorporate perceptions and interpretations that require acting upon. The decisions you make may be simple or more complex and you are likely to use a variety of data to come to a judgement. Subjective experience relates to how a person experiences their situation and is usually relayed through description. Interpretation may add further subjective data. An objective view, on the other hand, makes use of data that can be measured and recorded, such as vital signs and test results, for example (Hinchliff et al., 2008). Within clinical practice, both of these views are relevant and indeed valuable.

However, what reflection adds is the possibility of looking for threads of meaning running through, and possibly between, the information produced from these approaches. An analysis of these threads of meaning as additional processes helps to surface issues such as power, including lack of it, and how these relate to the situation. It is meaning that is not immediately obvious, and reflection endeavours to draw this out in order to read situations more accurately and to develop decision making and the effectiveness of practice. Reading the scenario of Natasha's A & E experience and thinking about the question at the end will help you to understand these processes further.

Scenario: Natasha's experience of under-age consent

*Natasha was near the end of the second year of her nurse preparation programme and working in an A & E unit. On this particular shift, a 15-year-old girl was brought in with a suspected **ectopic pregnancy**. She was adamant that she did not want her mother to know. Natasha recorded her vital signs of temperature, pulse, respirations and blood pressure, and noted that her pulse was elevated and her blood pressure was lower than was normal. Natasha started to develop a conversation with the patient while she undertook this task and asked her why she did not want her mother to know. The patient informed Natasha that she had always felt judged by her mother, who did not like her friends and was always criticising her. This would only confirm to her mother that she was 'no good', as she put it. She mostly stayed with friends and spent as little time at home as possible. The patient asked Natasha to call her boyfriend instead.*

After the patient had had an ultrasound scan, the obstetrician and gynaecological surgeon decided that the patient would need an operation. She was still adamant that she did not want her mother to know. Her boyfriend was not interested in staying, saying he would 'see her later'. The patient went to theatre without her mother knowing and with Natasha accompanying her. Natasha, only four years older, wondered about the sense of this.

continued . . .

Questions

- What are the main issues within this scenario?
- Who holds the power and in what way?
- What alternatives were available to the practitioners concerned?

There are outline answers to these questions at the end of the chapter.

Chapter summary

This chapter has illustrated a number of ways in which you can develop as a reflective practitioner. Through the examples and scenarios it has highlighted the importance of learning from mistakes and has offered opportunities for learning to challenge poor practice in ourselves and others. By continuing to use reflection to inform your practice, you will be able to recognise the connections between events and how you are progressing, as well as how issues such as power are important to the outcome of decisions. The importance of sharing your reflections in order to develop practice within the wider profession of nursing is continued in the next chapter, which looks at forms of reflecting with others.

Activities and scenarios: Brief outline answers

Activity 7.1: Reflection (page 91)

You might have identified that honesty from yourself and others is important to you so that both parties can be relied upon. You may also have found that doing as you would be done by is a central value for you, so that you can be trusted. You might have identified that you find unkindness difficult to bear because of the emotional distress it can cause. It is likely that you will have become aware of changes in your values and beliefs when entering your teenage years and when embarking on working life, and possibly parenthood. You might even have noticed changes when entering your nursing preparation programme. Changes are likely to have resulted from greater life experience modifying and altering value responses, although core values will still remain. These issues might relate to your practice in how you think about team working and your attitudes to both patients and colleagues.

Activity 7.2: Critical thinking (page 93)

Contributing factors that may have interfered with your decision making may range from tiredness and overwork to stress and lack of knowledge. Equally, not taking account of the patient's view may mean that interventions fail due to non-compliance. What you are likely to have tried to do afterwards was to rectify the decision and rebuild your self-esteem. However, without reflecting on the quality of the decision and the surrounding circumstances, not all the deficits might have been noticed and therefore only a partial solution may have been put in place. Equally, if you have not reflected you are likely to view the decision with shame and think less of yourself. Reflection helps to rebuild self-confidence and self-esteem. When considering how to make good decisions in response to your reflection you might have identified that including others in the decision-making processes could help to overcome stress and lack of knowledge. Equally, including the patient could also help to avoid non-compliance. You might also have thought about reflecting with others to develop your own decision-making skills.

Scenario: Pavlina's professional experience (pages 91–2)

Pavlina is likely to have learned that different professionals can work as a team. Pavlina is likely to have also learned the importance of policy and guidelines for informing practice. Her reflection with Gabriel has highlighted that she has been able to translate her new knowledge into explanations to reassure patients. During their reflection they might have considered the power relations between the different staff groups. They might also have considered whether consent was really informed when taken just before the procedure. The potential options for change that they might have thought about could include the following.

- The radiologists could visit inpatients on wards and give explanations and take consent in the morning. The attendance of outpatients for procedural appointments can be assumed to imply consent.
- Patient handover to ward staff could be undertaken in an office with checking of nursing observations and wound sites undertaken in the procedure room.

Pavlina is likely to have left this placement with a view of professionalism that is open to feedback and which is constantly reflecting to develop practice.

Scenario: Elsie's escapade (pages 93–4)

What contributed to practitioner fallibility in this scenario was an assumption that Elsie's behaviour was related solely to her confusion and that, because her observation recordings were normal, there was nothing wrong. It is easy to dismiss possible cues in such a way. What should have been done was to view the situation critically. This would have entailed asking a number of questions, such as the following.

- What might have contributed to Elsie ending up sitting on the grass?
- Is the way she is calling different from usual?
- What is triggering it?
- What calms her?

A thorough physical examination should have been carried out as there were no witnesses to how Elsie ended up sitting on the grass. If the nurses had started this, they might have been alerted by more signs, which would have given more impetus for the doctor to come and see Elsie as well. Other measurements, such as recording oxygen saturation and blood sugar, might also have been appropriate to ascertain why Elsie might have ended up sitting. It is likely that the practitioners will have been asked to review and justify their decision-making processes via a clinical incident form and through statements. Students involved in such situations would also be required to provide written testaments.

What might be learned from this situation is the need for assertive decision making and leadership that reads the cues from situations accurately. Continual assessment that focuses on the patient and does not rely only on monitoring devices is an essential part of this process. Recognising that a situation has changed comes partly from experience, but also through being open-minded and having a reflective attitude that does not accept circumstances at face value.

Scenario: Roger's near miss (page 96)

Roger learned that even with the correct checking procedures mistakes can still happen when there are earlier errors in a chain of events. He has learned to ensure that in his own practice documentation is carried out in a timely manner and the importance of delegation when the unit is busy.

Sarah and Roger both responded emotionally to the near miss with shock and anger aimed at the colleague who had put them in this position by not documenting correctly. When thinking about the incident they considered their options, although Roger's suggestion of asking the patient was viewed as not entirely reliable. It could also send a message that staff might not be competent. Sarah and Roger's behavioural responses were to ensure their own timely documentation when involved in drug administration.

The unit manager is likely to have undertaken some group reflection with the staff concerned and then developed this into some refresher training for all staff to ensure such an incident did not happen again. By taking an educative rather than a punitive approach, the unit manager is much more likely to enable the staff concerned to regain self-esteem and develop good practice. Another option would be to introduce regular clinical supervision opportunities for staff to be able to reflect on their own practice in a confidential environment.

Scenario: Natasha's experience of under-age consent (pages 97–8)

The main issues are the patient's clinical condition, which is serious, her request for confidentiality, the age of the patient, her mental competence and the rights of the mother. The clinical danger comes from the possibility of ectopic rupture, which can cause major haemorrhage and which requires operating on. Since the passing of the Gillick Law in 1985, doctors are required to assess the competency of under-age minors to make their own decisions. If the person is deemed to be competent and fully understands the facts of the situation, he or she may be deemed competent by the doctor to make the decision and to be able to give consent. However, it is for the doctor to decide whether the complexity of the decision is in keeping with the limits of consent and the person's competence.

The other alternatives available might have been to persuade the patient to tell her mother herself, or to allow a member of the team to do so, or to inform another member of the family who she felt able to talk to. Natasha needs to remember not to superimpose her subjective experience on to that of the patient. The objective data of the vital signs recording and the ultrasound have identified the clinical urgency and the patient's subjective experience has informed her decision.

Further reading

Johns, C (ed.) (2009) *Becoming a Reflective Practitioner*, 3rd edition. Chichester: Wiley-Blackwell.

This book will help you to gain an understanding of developing as a reflective practitioner in different contexts and through creative means.

Standing, M (2011) *Clinical Judgement and Decision-making for Nursing Students*. Exeter: Learning Matters.

This book offers a matrix model for decision making illustrated by case studies.

Useful website

www.nmc-uk.org/hearings (Nursing and Midwifery Council Fitness for Practice hearing outcomes)

Click on the hearing you want to look at and then on the outcomes for the detail of the case. Reading cases from the NMC website will help you to comprehend the significance of justifying your practice and the importance of continuing to reflect on it in order to ensure your effectiveness.

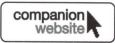
For further activities and other useful material, visit the companion website at
www.sagepub.co.uk/howatson-jones_reflective2e

Chapter 8
Guided reflection and reflecting with others

continued . . .

8.   People can trust the newly registered graduate nurse to gain their consent based on sound understanding in order to allow an informed choice prior to any intervention and that their rights in decision making and consent will be respected and upheld.

By the first progression point:

1.   Seeks consent prior to sharing confidential information outside of the professional care team, subject to agreed safeguarding and protection procedures.

Cluster: Organisational aspects of care

11.   People can trust the newly registered graduate nurse to safeguard children and adults from vulnerable situations and support and protect them from harm.

By the first progression point:

2.   Shares information with colleagues and seeks advice from appropriate sources where there is a concern or uncertainty.
3.   Uses support systems to recognise, manage and deal with own emotions.
12.   People can trust the newly registered graduate nurse to respond to their feedback and a wide range of other sources to learn, develop and improve services.

By the first progression point:

1.   Responds appropriately to compliments and comments.

Chapter aims

After reading this chapter you will be able to:

*   identify ways of dealing with the emotional residues of caring work;
*   reflect in a group as part of action learning;
*   reflect with other professionals;
*   define guided reflection;
*   understand clinical supervision frameworks and models.

Example story

Sally was in the second year of her nurse preparation programme and on a placement at a hospice. She had been very nervous about going there as she was not sure whether she would be able to cope with this type of nursing. She imagined that all the patients would be dying and that it would be a very depressing place to work. She was surprised to find that there was a variety of patients and that there was a cheerful atmosphere. The nurses worked efficiently but made sure that they also gave a lot of time to the patients. Sharon, Sally's mentor, assigned Amanda – a lady who had been treated for breast cancer but who now had lung and bony **metastases** – for Sally to look after over a number of shifts.

Sally found that she and Amanda had many things in common, even though Amanda was ten years older than her. Amanda used to be a dancer, but when she became ill the treatments exhausted her too much to continue. Sally loved salsa dancing and went out most weekends to a salsa bar with her friends. She told Amanda about some of their escapades, which made her laugh. As Amanda weakened, Sally became increasingly involved in her personal care. On Sally's last placement shift she went into Amanda's room and found her breathing had changed. Sharon told her that this was the last stage before imminent death and encouraged Sally to stay with Amanda so she would not be alone, as she had no family nearby. Sharon felt that Sally was ready for this last important care that she could offer Amanda. Sally wanted to do this. Amanda died peacefully three hours later.

Sharon came in to help Sally prepare Amanda and to give her a chance to talk about this last stage of nursing. Sally said she could understand now why nurses said they found this type of nursing satisfying. She told Sharon how privileged she felt to be there at the end, supporting Amanda through this difficult phase. As they prepared Amanda, Sharon also asked Sally to describe the changes she had witnessed in Amanda as she approached death and afterwards. Sharon's purpose for doing this was twofold. First, it would help Sally to recognise signs and stages of death, and, second, it would help her to disengage from emotional attachment with Amanda so she could leave the shift composed. Through the process of preparation Sally felt that they had been respectful of Amanda and she left the shift feeling sad but also satisfied with her care.

Back at the university, Sally was kept busy with thinking about assignments and completing her course work. It was a few weeks later when Sally was sharing the practice experience with other students on her programme during a class that she realised how profoundly this experience had affected her. As the tutor helped the group to reflect on their experiences, she encouraged them to explore and analyse their responses and decisions, and what sense they were making of what was happening at the time and afterwards. Sally realised that her reaction to the situation stemmed from the emotional residues that this event had left behind. She had been close to Amanda and was sad to have that connection broken. She also felt concern about what Amanda might have been feeling at the end. Sally had made use of touch to communicate her concern and talked quietly to Amanda. Ann, one of the class members, suggested that Sally and Sharon might have been trying to control the situation, as Amanda had no way of telling them whether she wanted this type of communication or not.

Sally was struck by the fact that it was difficult to determine what patients wanted during end of life care, as beyond a certain point nursing was based on nurses' assumptions and experience, and not necessarily upon patients' wishes. This could potentially make the experience extremely variable for the person if the nurses' assumptions were wrong. Sally thought about conversations she had overheard, talking about patients having a difficult death because they would not 'let go'. Sally wondered about the accuracy of such judgements. This was a challenging thought for Sally as she considered the possibilities of this care experience. The process of reflection had moved her from an emotional position to thinking about her practice.

Introduction

The example above is offered to help illustrate how reflective questioning from others can add depth to reflection and develop a wider understanding. Good facilitation helps to contain the anxiety that might surround such a process. As you progress through your nurse preparation programme, so opportunities to learn from the experience of others also arise. This is especially true of the interprofessional learning activities that form part of the preparation programme and when working with others in practice.

This chapter will consider how guided reflection can deepen your understanding and analysis of situations, experiences and decisions, and how reflecting with others can offer support. Within this also lies a discussion of the increasing importance of skilful supervision within modern healthcare to make sense of changing roles. The chapter builds on the previous ones by drawing on different professional cultures and styles of guided reflection to identify how reflection, and forms thereof, are applicable across a growing range of professions, and how increased inter-professional working and learning contributes to shared reflective opportunities. The chapter identifies the spaces that exist between practitioners and how these might be facilitated to be compelling to reflective learning and personal development, in order to develop better under-standings of practice.

Ways of dealing with the emotional residues of caring work

Caring work inevitably leaves some emotional imprints. When reflecting, actions and rela-tionships are scrutinised and critiqued, and your personal identity comes into prominence as you develop. Examining an event means cultural, social, historical and psychological aspects are considered when giving an account (van Boven et al., 2003), for example what led up to the event, what particular groups of people were involved and their perspectives, and how people might be feeling. Learning provokes anxiety by admitting uncertainty and the need to shift thinking. Undertake Activity 8.1 using the example at the start to apply these ideas, in order to help develop your understanding.

Activity 8.1   *Critical thinking*

Read the example at the start of the chapter again. Now examine what you perceive are the main cultural, historical and psychological aspects of the situation for those involved. Are these different for the various people; and, if you think so, how are they different? Now imagine yourself in Sally's place. Are your perceptions the same or have they changed? If so, how have they changed and is there a relationship with the stage of preparation you are at?

There is an outline answer to this activity at the end of the chapter.

When undertaking this activity you might have been challenged to confront your views and fears about nursing a dying person. You might have questioned whether you were 'up to it'. You might have thought about situations that proved that this might be a problem for you. Shame is often experienced in the workplace and may occur within supervisory relationships (Lynch et al., 2008). For example, if you get something wrong, you may worry that your mentor thinks less of you as a person and as a nurse. Anxiety can affect your confidence and make you prone to mistakes that you would not normally make. Relationships that are supportive and secure enough to allow exploration of thoughts and feelings can provide a form of containment for anxiety (Holmes, 2005). Building a good relationship with your mentor is a joint venture and responsibility. Consider the following scenario and answer the question at the end to help you think about this.

Scenario: Veronica's first day on a new placement

Veronica was in the first year of her mental health nurse preparation programme and today was the first day of her placement with the community mental health nurses. She was excited about this placement because she thought the community might be somewhere where she would like to work in the future. She met Greg, her mentor, at the community nurses' base. Greg welcomed Veronica and introduced her to other members of the team. He explained who people were and how things worked. He also filled her in on what they would be doing that day. Their first visit was to see Harry, a 65-year-old man who lived alone. Veronica was taken aback by the state of his home. There were newspapers piled up everywhere and what appeared to be bags of rubbish. The smell was overpowering. Greg checked that Harry was taking his medication and had a chat with him and then they left. The morning continued to be busy, but at lunchtime Greg sat down with Veronica and asked her if she was all right as he had picked up on her reaction when they visited Harry. Veronica shared her feelings of shock that anybody would want to live like that. She asked Greg how Harry could get into such a state. Greg asked her to think about some of the ways she tried to maintain control in her own life. They then reflected on some of the potential causes of Harry's behaviour and how to support him. Veronica went home that day with a different perspective of community mental health nursing, but she also felt that Greg had supported her without making her feel silly.

Questions
- What are the main issues in this scenario?
- In what other ways could Greg further support Veronica?
- What else could Veronica do to enhance her understanding?

There are outline answers to these questions at the end of the chapter.

This scenario will have helped you to critically review what is going on in situations that you might experience as difficult. Taking ownership of the situation and looking for solutions can be challenging. Critically examining events may also challenge your accepted identity by highlighting weaknesses you may not have been aware of. Supported self-awareness helps to hold the tension of confronted identity and facilitate reconstructions that lead to learning and change (Lindsay, 2006). Facilitating such learning is a key part of your mentor's role, but being open to developing insight is a key part of yours. We proceed now to consider how reflecting in a group can help to develop such critical awareness and how this might be sustained through the process of action learning.

Reflecting in a group as part of action learning

Developmental journeys are made up of stories, some of which may be care stories and some of which relate to the practitioner (Bishop, 2007). Action learning is a process that reflects on real-life situations with a group of practitioners in order to develop problem solving and knowledge. It draws together knowledge, experiential learning and creativity to come to new solutions. The importance is the spiral of continuity, which takes forward learning and transforms it into action. Group involvement is vital for achieving depth of reflection and breadth of consideration of potential solutions, and for encouragement and support. The roles of various group members are as follows.

The presenter   proposes an issue and needs to be able to present it in such a way that group members can understand it, so that the message is communicated succinctly. The presenter also needs to be open to feedback and be able to explain the action plan they are taking forward, to retain ownership of the problem.

Group members   ask questions to clarify the problem and offer reflective insights to possible surrounding factors and other ways of viewing the situation. They discuss the merits of potential solutions and reflect on possible consequences that might arise from these, to enable an informed choice to be made. They remain focused on the issue at hand.

The facilitator   attends and observes the group process, adding challenge, reflective insights and support as required. The facilitator summarises the learning and actions at key stages of the group process, to keep things on track.

Confidentiality is a founding principle of such group working; without trusting that what is discussed will be kept within the group, it will be difficult for group members to share fully. Consequently, when such groups are set up they will often start with a contracting exercise in which the group agree on the rules for engagement and individual and group responsibilities. Confidentiality is a fundamental rule within such a contract. Being a group member means giving a commitment not only to keep discussions confidential, but also to demonstrate commitment to the group through attendance and contribution to the discussions. This helps to demonstrate respect for the value of working together. Sitting things out means that the learning environment required for individuals and the group to learn is not sustained.

The purpose of group reflection is to consolidate and develop professional knowledge and practice. Connections with mentorship and preceptorship draw on ideas of the development of the *professional craft* (Titchen et al., 2004: 108), which relates to you as a practitioner and how you engage with developing your knowledge and skills base. Mentorship and preceptorship are ways that others help to facilitate your development of nursing knowledge, but it is through actively learning with others that you are able to consolidate this knowledge, recognising your unique contribution, and expanding the skills base and confidence in your performance. Read the following scenario on the craft of nursing to develop your understanding of what this means.

Scenario: Anita's administration of an injection

Anita is an experienced staff nurse you are working with, but not your mentor. She has been a qualified nurse for 20 years and has worked on the unit you are on for 10 years. Today she has asked you to come and observe her administering an injection in order to develop your learning of this technique. Anita begins by going to explain to Betty (the patient) what she has planned, and to gain her consent. Betty does not really like needles. Anita returns to the clinical room with Betty's drug chart and checks it carefully, washes her hands and starts to gather the necessary equipment together. All the while she is explaining to you what she is doing and why, and asking you questions. She checks the drug ampoule and carefully draws up the drug with no spillage and little air being introduced into the syringe. She expels any air bubbles carefully into the vial to avoid drug spray. When you both arrive at Betty's bedside, Anita asks you to talk quietly to Betty and hold her hand while she prepares the area for injection. With swift, smooth, deft movements Anita swabs the skin, inserts the needle, injects the drug and removes the needle again, pressing slightly to stem any leakage and reassuring Betty calmly. Betty has hardly noticed the injection. This whole episode has taken less than 10 minutes.

You contrast Anita's fluidity with your own clumsy technique when administering your first injection. Skin is tougher than appears in this exemplar, so the efficiency of Anita's movements must be related to her expertise. The next time, you observe Anita much more closely in order to analyse what she is adding. You note her ease of communication, which relaxes the patient and which immediately makes the insertion of the needle easier. This first step appears crucial to the whole proceedings and makes the procedure less task-orientated and more patient-focused. You observe the coordination occurring between Anita's swabbing of the skin and insertion and withdrawal of the needle, and the attention that Anita gives to the detail of her patient's reaction and physical consequences. Patient comfort and procedural efficiency are both important.

Within this example Anita has developed fluidity from undertaking the procedure many times and from the slight adjustments she has learned each time in how a patient moves, responds and perhaps even flinches. The procedure has become second nature: she does not need to think about it and is able to explain and 'do' at the same time. This illustrates that the knowledge has become embedded (Sennett, 2008). However, Anita's prime focus is not the 'task' but the person. How she communicates with the patient is implicated as much in the skill she exhibits. Identifying how your practice interfaces with others is an important part of developing craft knowledge, by helping to highlight what is special to the nursing role and how others can contribute to developing this knowledge in other ways. We proceed now to consider the value of reflection with other professionals.

Reflecting with other professionals

Following the Darzi Report, the quality agenda is focused on developing the whole workforce to provide high-quality care (DH, 2008a) based on principles of quality, patient-centredness, flexibility, valuing people, clinical relevance and promoting lifelong learning (DH, 2008b). Boundaries are becoming blurred and teaching, learning and supervision opportunities arise for the novice as well as the expert practitioner as assistant roles expand. Reflection is not just about what has been learned, but about how the professional is changing. This is of particular significance when growing as a professional and how you develop reflective questions. As roles change and new ways of thinking become apparent, the implications for you as a growing professional are also important. Reflecting with other professionals can help to put this into perspective.

Completing Activity 8.2 will help you to find ways of doing this.

Activity 8.2 — *Reflection*

- Think back to your last few placements and consider where your practice interfaced with that of other professionals. Write a list of all the professions you have identified. Now consider what opportunities there might have been within these areas to share practice and develop learning.
- Now think about your university programme and list any other professionals that you learn with. Consider what opportunities there might be to share practice and develop learning.
- Review your findings and draw up an action plan for how you might be able to develop or take advantage of reflecting with other professionals. Identify what your objectives for doing so might be by drafting some reflective questions.

If you are an experienced practitioner, consider how you can develop opportunities for learning from other professionals for students and for yourself.

There is an outline answer to this activity at the end of the chapter.

The answers that you might have found when undertaking this activity enable you to exert some agency in your own learning and proactively plan how you can expand your knowledge of other professions and share practice. The interprofessional approach is important to open up possibilities and thereby enhance practice. However, for the novice this may be difficult and, where there are tensions between different professional groups, the process may be better supported by inclusion of a guide who can facilitate reflection. We proceed now to consider the role of guided reflection.

Guided reflection

Guided reflection is defined as reflection that, through the questioning and insights of another more experienced practitioner, can get beneath the surface of experience. The guide helps the practitioner to reveal self-deceptions and limits to vision, as well as supplying support and encouragement to deepen learning (Johns, 2010). In this way it becomes possible to peel back layers of what may initially be perceived as routine practice to reach the essence of deeper learning underneath, much as peeling back the layers of an onion intensifies the chemical effects of aroma. Because, during guided reflection, the practitioner is expected to confront self-deceptions and distortions within their reflecting, it is important that facilitation is supportive and well thought out. This is why an experienced and qualified person is required.

Facilitating containment involves setting clear boundaries and providing structure so that people do not lose themselves, or what they are supposed to be doing (Thorndycraft and McCabe, 2008). The following case study is offered to help illustrate how guided reflection might be used to reflect on a critical incident to provide the support required to deal with the emotional residues, as well as to develop reflective learning.

Pat's experience of sudden death

Pat was in the third year of her nurse preparation programme working in A & E. She was working on the night shift on this particular day. It was a busy Friday night and the emergency phone rang with a message to say that there had been a serious accident and seven teenagers were being brought in with severe injuries. They had been travelling in one car and the driver had been distracted and hit the slip ramp wall. Two of the teenagers were pronounced dead on arrival in A & E and the other five required immediate surgery. Pat helped with laying out the two who had died because their relatives were coming. She was struck by how peaceful they looked, just as if they were asleep. She went home the next morning feeling rather disturbed by this incident. Pat's mentor, Simon, was aware that this was likely to have been a difficult experience for Pat and met with her at the start of the following night shift. He explained that they had 20 minutes and explored with Pat how she felt about the experience. Pat told Simon she had found it disturbing. They explored the reasons for this. Pat had children of her own close to the age of the teenagers. She could imagine the pain of their parents. It also made her confront her own mortality and how life could be snuffed out in a moment. Simon helped her to see that she had completed a valuable nursing role in preparing the two teenagers to be seen by their parents and for being a comforting presence.

This case study has demonstrated the importance of guided reflection after critical incidents such as might occur in sudden death. However, guided reflection is equally important for reflecting on everyday practice in order to review what you do and how to improve it. Clinical supervision is a form of guided reflection that can enable you to do this. The following section explains what clinical supervision is, what it is not, and some of the models and frameworks that are used.

Clinical supervision frameworks

Clinical supervision is a practice-focused relationship with a professional that enables you to work through emotionally charged situations to release stress, and explore and reflect on your work, in order to gain constructive feedback and affirmation of effective practice. The experienced professional is the supervisor and the person reflecting is the supervisee. Clinical supervision is relevant because it connects with various forms of support and has a role within quality agendas for practice (Morton-Cooper and Palmer, 2000). Clinical supervision is a form of experiential learning that supports reflective examination of practice and planning of development (Milne, 2009).

Variations on using clinical supervision include autobiographical reports from colleagues, vignettes from supervisee and supervisor, and educational input; and networking with other disciplines to share supervisors provides an enriching influence on the process (Howatson-Jones, 2003). These variations have relevance to the facilitation and the tasks of supervision. Support and clarity of boundaries of responsibility, which make professionals think about their self-concept as practitioners in such contexts, are crucial to achieve learning and avoid doing harm through the clinical supervision process (Phelan et al., 2006). Careful planning of objectives and goals, and working more creatively through the harnessing of technology such as a wiki, or using existing forums such as progress meetings for the student and ward meetings for the more experienced practitioner, to provide clarification, are all ways considered in how implementation might be broadened. The managerial role in terms of actual supervision and of caring for the well-being of the workforce is crucial to establishing effective supervision that enables practitioners of all abilities and stages of progression to learn and feel good about themselves (van Ooijen, 2003). When considering your first qualified role, one of the provisions you might want to think about is whether the organisation you are applying to offers clinical supervision to its staff.

The NMC (2006) identifies clinical supervision as being important, and asserts these principles.

- Clinical supervision supports practice.
- Clinical supervision is a practice-focused relationship.
- Clinical supervision should be developed according to local need and circumstances.
- Ground rules should be agreed to support openness and transparency.
- Every practitioner should have access.
- There should be preparation for supervisors.
- Evaluation of clinical supervision should take place to determine influence on care.

But clinical supervision is only as effective as the ability of the practitioner to be self-aware, and to have some insight into their own feelings and behaviours. Key stages of the reflective process within clinical supervision include the following.

- **Self-awareness**   the process of getting to know feelings, attitudes and values.
- **Description**   the ability to recognise and recollect key events.
- **Critical analysis**   examining components, and challenging assumptions and exploring alternatives.

- **Synthesis**   integration of new knowledge and identifying action.
- **Evaluation**   making judgements about the value of the experience.

Self-awareness is about the kind of relationship you have with yourself. For example, are you always critical of yourself, or too demanding in your expectations, or not demanding enough? Maybe there are times when your appraisal of yourself might not be accurate or realistic. For example, you might think that you know how to do something because you have completed the task in simulation, without realising that because patients vary, your practice in the initial stages will be supervised by someone more experienced. This will happen no matter how competent you feel. Expectations and self-appraisal are all implicated in the type of behaviours we exhibit, and how open to feedback we might, or might not, be. The skills and attributes needed for engaging with, and getting the most out of, clinical supervision include: communication skills, reflective ability, honesty and being open to feedback.

There are a number of models of clinical supervision. These include calling on an expert facilitator who has expertise in the problem area and can offer some solutions; one-to-one supervision where the individual meets with the supervisor alone; group supervision where a number of people meet with a supervisor; or using a supervisor from another discipline. Consideration of the model for supervision depends on whether the issue for discussion requires an expert, whether peer discussion could benefit all parties, whether a group holds similar concerns or whether an individual requires support, or whether the issue is too sensitive to be aired in a group setting. Whichever is chosen, it is important to be clear about the aims of clinical supervision sessions.

Proctor (1986, cited in Hawkins and Shohet, 1989, p42) devised a framework that drew together the managerial, educative and support functions of clinical supervision. These are interpreted as follows.

1. **Normative**
   (a) Managerial function concerned with safe practice/developing standards.
   (b) Ensures adherence to guidelines.
   (c) Talking to more experienced practitioner assists supervisee to work within these guidelines and meet standards.

2. **Educational**
   (a) Reflection and exploration.
   (b) Enables supervisee to recognise strengths and weaknesses to develop.
   (c) Relates theory to practice in a critical way.

3. **Restorative**
   (a) Supportive function of responding.
   (b) Helps to understand how emotional involvement affects practice.
   (c) Enables nurses to deal with their own reactions.
   (d) Provides a workforce that can deal with critical incidents/problems.

Another framework is offered by van Ooijen (2003), which views getting the most out of clinical supervision as a developmental journey, as illustrated in Figure 8.1. The starting point is as a novice in the use and understanding of clinical supervision, but as competence and knowledge

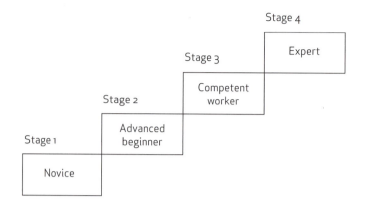

Figure 8.1: Developmental framework
Published in van Ooijen, E (2003) *Clinical Supervision Made Easy*. Elsevier. Used with permission.

increase, so practitioners start to become more independent in their thinking – which continues to grow with increasing expertise when engaging with clinical supervision.

At the start of the journey, supervisees are highly motivated but lack insight and experience. As they progress to the next stage, they oscillate between being dependent on the supervisor and becoming more autonomous. At the stage after this, the supervisees have more confidence in their judgements, and at the end they act autonomously, with the supervision process becoming two-way in terms of reflective learning.

Clinical supervision, as noted at the start, offers the opportunity to develop reflective learning and deal with the emotional residues of caring work. According to Faugier and Butterworth (1994), clinical supervision is:

- sharing practice-based issues in confidence;
- getting feedback and guidance;
- developing professional knowledge through reflection;
- letting off steam;
- acknowledging feelings;
- feeling valued through supervisory support.

What clinical supervision is *not* is:

- complaining;
- unstructured sharing of events;
- personal/family matters;
- being told what to do;
- disciplinary issues;
- other colleagues' performance.

Undertaking Activity 8.3 will help you to apply these ideas in order to identify some suitable topics to bring to clinical supervision.

Activity 8.3 *Critical thinking*

Spend a little time thinking of topics that you think would be suitable to take to a clinical supervision session. Make a list so that you can reconsider how these might change during your working week. You can develop this further by choosing a trusted peer to offer peer supervision.

There is an outline answer to this activity at the end of the chapter.

It is important to reflect on a suitable topic well before a clinical supervision session in order to prioritise what is significant for your learning. According to Driscoll (2007), a clinical supervision session involves:

- **preparation**: reflecting on the topic you plan to bring;
- **settling in**: the clinical supervisor will help you to relax;
- **down to business**: you will be asked to present your issue concisely;
- **clarification and summarising**: the supervisor will clarify what is important;
- **closure**: the supervisor closes the session with action planning.

As you will have noticed, clinical supervision is focused on your learning through the topics that you bring. It is also time that is dedicated to you and therefore something that is very valuable and affirming. Making regular use of it as a healthcare practitioner can really help you to grow.

Chapter summary

This chapter has looked at a number of different reflective frameworks and ways of reflecting with others. The importance of others in stimulating the breadth of reflective knowledge has been emphasised because nursing interfaces with so many professions and this can enrich reflective processes. Through the examples and case studies you have been given an illustration of possible applications, with the activities offering you some guidance on identifying how you might proceed to incorporate some of these forms of reflection into your own practice and learning. How you start to record your reflections and write reflectively as another form of development is explored in the next chapter.

Activities and scenarios: Brief outline answers

Activity 8.1: Critical thinking (page 104)

Death, with the rituals that may accompany it, and how people feel about it, has many different cultural meanings. These may relate to belief systems as well as to personal values. Belief systems may be religious as well as historically embedded in a culture. For the nurse, belief rituals and psychological aspects are the focus. In the example, cultural meaning for Sharon lies in her belief that people should not die alone. Historically, this has been a common value in nursing. Sally followed this direction because of the psychological, emotional bond she had developed with Amanda. Sally is more emotionally bound to the situation than Sharon is. But Sharon is aware of the psychological residues for Sally and offers support, creating an encouraging culture for learning. It is hard to know what Amanda would have wanted, although there might have been some historical clues leading up to the event. For example, she might have preferred a relative or friend to be with her and this might have been evident through her conversations about her life when she talked to Sally earlier on.

If you are in the early stages of your nurse preparation programme, the psychological aspects might be the most prominent for you, depending on your history and whether you have had many dealings with death before. If you are more experienced, you will have been exposed for longer to the culture of nursing and will have developed coping mechanisms to help you deal with psychological feelings. If you are very experienced like Sharon, your history as a nurse will determine what you see as important, how you react and what kind of cultures you create.

Activity 8.2: Reflection (page 108)

You might have identified placements such as radiology, offering an interface with radiographers; rehabilitation areas, providing access to physiotherapists, occupational therapists and social workers; theatres, enabling connection with operating department practitioners; and women's health and day surgery arenas, offering an interface with midwifery. Equally, during your sampling weeks you will have access to other professionals such as those working with mental health and learning disabilities. All of these offer opportunities for reflecting with others through meetings, especially multi-disciplinary meetings, reflective learning groups and case conferences. Equally, at university you may be involved in some joint learning with other health and social care students, and this will often involve some element of reflection on developing professional identity and the contribution from different professions. Your action plan might have identified how to arrange to become involved in some of the activities identified above the next time you are on placement. You might also have included thinking in more detail about who your practice has interfaced with and what you have learned when talking in the classroom. Your initial reflective questions might be as follows.

* How does this profession's priorities interface with those of nurses?
* What, as a nurse practitioner, can I learn about this profession?

As an experienced practitioner you might have considered arranging opportunities for students to spend the day with professionals allied to your area. You might also consider arranging for these professionals to undertake some teaching sessions in your area to share practice.

Activity 8.3: Critical thinking (page 113)

The kind of topics that you might have thought about could include:

* professional issues;
* exploring learning and development options;
* work-related interpersonal relations;
* ethical/legal issues;
* work experiences, both positive and negative;
* skills development;
* managerial development.

You may have identified some new ideas when reflecting with your trusted peer and might have been open to their suggestions because you trusted them. However, while such guided reflection is useful for opening up your critical thinking you will need an experienced guide to reach any depth.

Scenario: Veronica's first day on a new placement (page 105)

The first issue in the scenario is the first impression that Greg's welcome for Veronica has given. This first impression has stayed with her, making her feel valued and supported, and counteracting the anxiety of the visit to Harry. The second issue is Veronica's shock at Harry's behaviour, which clearly is at odds with Veronica's values and beliefs. Greg could explore these further with her. Greg could further support Veronica by sharing his thinking and decision making about Harry with her. Veronica could enhance her understanding by sourcing information in the mental health literature about the reasons for such behaviours.

Further reading

Higgs, J, Richardson, B and Abrandt Dahlgren, M (eds) (2004) *Developing Practice Knowledge for Health Professionals*. Edinburgh: Butterworth Heinemann.

This book will help you to understand how craft knowledge develops and how this relates to different forms of knowledge.

Johns, C (2010) *Guided Reflection: A narrative approach to advancing professional practice*, 2nd edition. Chichester: Wiley-Blackwell.

This book explains guided reflection through a number of exemplars and the author's practice.

Milne, D (2009) *Evidence-based Clinical Supervision: Principles and practice*. Oxford: British Psychological Society and Blackwell.

This book presents that evidence base for using clinical supervision techniques and is especially useful for experienced practitioners in developing their practice.

van Ooijen, E (2003) *Clinical Supervision Made Easy*. Edinburgh: Churchill Livingstone.

This book explains clinical supervision in a way that is easy to understand.

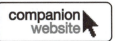

For further activities and other useful material, visit the companion website at
www.sagepub.co.uk/howatson-jones_reflective2e

Chapter 9
Reflective writing

continued . . .

By the second progression point:

6. Uses strategies to enhance communication and remove barriers to effective communication, minimising risk to people from lack of or poor communication.
7. People can trust the newly registered graduate nurse to protect and keep as confidential all information relating to them.

By the first progression point:

2. Protects and treats information as confidential except where sharing information is required for the purposes of safeguarding and public protection.
3. Applies the principles of data protection.

Cluster: Organisational aspects of care

12. People can trust the newly registered graduate nurse to respond to their feedback and a wide range of other sources to learn, develop and improve services.

By the first progression point:

1. Responds appropriately to compliments and comments.

By the second progression point:

3. Uses supervision and other forms of reflective learning to make effective use of feedback.
18. People can trust a newly registered graduate nurse to enhance the safety of service users and identify and actively manage risk and uncertainty in relation to people, the environment, self and others.

By the first progression point:

6. Knows and accepts own responsibilities and takes appropriate action.

Chapter aims

After reading this chapter you will be able to:

- define writing reflectively;
- understand the principles of confidentiality and reflective writing;
- undertake personal reflective writing, such as keeping a reflective journal;
- undertake personal development planning;
- write reflectively in assignments as appropriate;
- record guided reflection.

Example story

Khalid was in the first year of his nurse preparation programme. As part of his professional development he was required to keep a reflective log of his professional and academic development. One of his assignments also required him to reflect on his first practice experience and write this up within the assignment.

Khalid began logging how he felt when starting his nursing course. He also described the activities and classes he had completed and how he felt he had managed these. As time went on and the pressure of the programme took over, Khalid forgot to log his experiences. He discussed his practice experience with his peers and what it had been like, but did not record anything. As the submission date for his assignment drew nearer Khalid started to think about what he would write. He found his logged notes and started to compose a descriptive account of his experiences. He emailed the first draft to his tutor.

Khalid's tutor responded by saying that, although his work showed how Khalid felt about things, there was no reflective analysis of what he had learned or how he was developing. Khalid realised that reflective writing was more than just describing what he had done or how he felt and not as easy as he had at first thought it to be. He was not used to analysing why he felt the way he did, or scrutinising his own actions. However, when he spoke with his peers Khalid became aware that he was critiquing other people's actions. Khalid decided he would try to examine his own actions by having a critical conversation with himself.

Back at his home Khalid began by asking himself questions about what had happened, why it was important and what he thought about it now. He then returned to the issue, using the 'so what' question (see the discussion of Driscoll's reflective cycle in Chapter 4). Structuring his reflection more rigorously in this way helped Khalid to start writing in a more analytical way. He revisited his early logs and began reworking them in a similar way as he revisited the events.

By adopting this more in-depth approach to reviewing his placement experience, Khalid was able to write about how what he had learned could be developed further. He connected the main points he was making with some of what he had learned on the programme and some recent reading he had completed, as well as literature about reflection. Khalid was pleased to achieve a mark of 70 per cent in his assignment.

Introduction

Learning to write reflectively will equip you with the relevant ethical and analytical ability to benefit from your practice experiences. To do this you will need to look back on significant incidents and examine surrounding concepts and analysis of them. This chapter will explore the purpose of reflective writing in relation to the standards of proficiency required by nursing regulators. You will be introduced to a variety of techniques and encouraged to try out some different exercises to help to develop this skill. In particular, you will be invited to begin personal development planning related to your reflective log. How to write reflectively in assignments is also considered.

Writing reflectively

Writing about your experiences will help you to make sense of them so that your understanding lasts and contributes to your lifelong learning. Reflection about experiences may be articulated in different ways when you are speaking or writing about them. Speaking about situations tends to be exploratory as your thought is put into words. However, writing about the circumstances may sometimes be subject to concerns with the presentation and the scrutiny of an invisible audience. It is important, when starting out to write reflectively, that concerns about who might read it are reduced, in order for you to be able to be truly honest and authentic in your reflective evaluation and writing about your experience. Bolton (2010) suggests that, just like Alice in Wonderland, it is important to be open to uncertainty and new experience in playful ways. In other words, to go *through the mirror* and see where it takes you (Bolton, 2010, p69). Writing in this way demands breadth and depth, and a commitment to explore and not to be afraid of what you might find out. Starting such a writing journey means writing in formative and unfinished ways, capturing your deepest thoughts and feelings as they start to surface. Consider the following examples of reflective writing from the student nurse and ward manager perspective, and then answer the questions in Activity 9.1.

Student reflection example

I am a student nurse (my name is Maria) on a child nursing preparation programme and am having difficulties with my placement ward manager. I was working a shift and forgot to pass on a message to the parents of a child I was looking after. The next day the ward manager, Rachel, told me off at handover. I feel persecuted, bullied and very upset. This is compromising my learning. I spoke to the link tutor, Martin, who arranged a meeting with Rachel and me. I know other students have also complained about this ward. The meeting with Martin and Rachel helped to clarify our expectations of each other. In particular it made me think about the importance of carrying out duties that have been delegated to me. But I am still unsure whether Rachel will fulfil her commitment to discuss concerns in private. I still feel on edge. This means that I am focused on not getting things wrong. As a consequence I am reluctant to try out new things and am learning less than my colleagues. Perhaps I am being over-sensitive, but I do feel that this incident has highlighted the kind of manager I do not want to be. I think it is better to talk privately to someone if I have an issue with them because issues can be aired properly. This also allows the opportunity to manage emotions before facing others. If this happened to me again I would ask the manager to take me somewhere private. But I will also keep a notebook for noting down essential tasks to help me to remember.

Practitioner reflection example

I am Rachel, a ward manager of a busy children's ward in an acute hospital. The ward was busy when I got a phone call from a child's parents complaining that they had not been told about a home visit that the physiotherapist was trying to arrange. When I asked the child's nurse she told me that Maria had been asked to tell them the date yesterday. I saw Maria at handover and asked her crossly why she had not passed on this message. I could see by the look on her face that I had upset her, but was too busy with ward business to do anything about it. Since then I have met with Martin, the link tutor, and Maria and agreed to discuss future concerns in private. Reflecting on this now I realise the impact telling Maria off in public is likely to have had and my responsibilities. I am sure she felt embarrassed and angry. I know I felt these emotions later about myself. I am the one in a position of power and am responsible for the learning environment of the ward as a placement area. Maria is likely to have learned how not to communicate concerns about performance. My behaviour has probably created a barrier to her learning because she may be frightened of being corrected by me again. I know my behaviour was sparked in part because of my worries about the skill mix on the ward and how short staffed we are. I seem to have to be everywhere at the moment. But that is no excuse as I am responsible. Thinking now about my communication with Maria, I could have spoken to her afterwards and apologised to show her we are all human. I could also have asked her how her learning was developing. I need to have greater control of my own emotions in order to help contain those of others. I clearly need to find a way to vent some of the stress I am feeling. I think I will seek some clinical supervision to help me with this. I will also arrange another meeting with Maria to apologise and find out how she feels she is progressing. I will give her the option to have Martin there if she wishes. In future I will make sure that performance issues are discussed privately with the person concerned.

Activity 9.1   *Reflection*

After reading the two examples of early reflective writing above, answer the following questions.

- What is Maria's focus for reflection?
- What is Rachel's focus for reflection?
- Are any further actions planned?
- If you were either Maria or Rachel, how could you add depth to the reflection?

There are outline answers to these questions at the end of the chapter.

There are many reasons for undertaking reflective writing. These include:

- to log and record personal and professional experience and development;
- to help make sense of emotionally charged situations;
- to record other forms of reflection, such as guided reflection;
- to identify and plan career progression;
- to provide evidence of learning;
- to fulfil assignment requirements;
- for your own interest.

Reasons for reflective writing may vary, but the result is beginning to feel more empowered as you take control of your own development and learning, and come to a more positive view of difficult situations. However, the actual process can be emotionally demanding in what it reveals about you as a person and perhaps about others too. Read the following scenario to consider what opportunity it presents for reflective writing.

Scenario: Faheed's experience of group cultural differences

Faheed was in the first year of his mental nurse preparation programme. His peer group at university comprised a diverse range of students from a variety of backgrounds and different professional pathways. They were studying a collaborative module that required them to develop patches of writing reflecting on professional values. They worked on these in groups and presented their writing to the class for peer feedback at the development stage.

Faheed recognised that there were problems with group dynamics when they were at a break and some people started complaining about the task and having to learn with other pathway students. Faheed spoke up, saying how important it was for professions to understand each other and work together for the good of the patient. He related a personal example of a family member recovering from serious injury because of different professions working together. The group returned to the class and task with fresh enthusiasm.

Question
- What learning might Faheed take from this situation?

There is an outline answer to this question at the end of the chapter.

Ehrmann (2005) identifies that disruptive and aggressive behaviours arise from power struggles and a sense of competitiveness, and may result in a failure to control self in practice, which has implications for patients and staff. Team relations in any situation are partly influenced by the personalities, psychological states and cultures of the people involved. Xu and Davidhizar (2005) suggest that there are cultural differences in communication patterns that can lead to misinterpretations and breakdowns. Western and European culture follows an individualistic pattern, while eastern and African cultures favour group patterns. Students sometimes feel dis-empowered and reluctant to share their needs for fear of discrimination (Dalton, 2005). When faced by a dominant group in the classroom, it might appear difficult to have your voice heard. If others' responses are not encouraging it is easy to become discouraged and silenced.

Equally, however, it will be necessary for people from different cultures to learn to adapt to each other in order to communicate adequately for patient care. Part of the learning process is to bridge these divides and develop opportunities. Further development can be achieved by continued reflection on what is happening and potential reasons why, and by considering alternatives. Writing reflectively will help you to deal with these types of situations and with the implementation of ideas. This is one way of gaining **empowerment** within such situations. However, as our experiences inevitably involve others too, it is important to recognise within reflective writing personal responsibility and accountability to maintain the anonymity and confidentiality of others. We proceed to consider this in the next section.

The principles of confidentiality in reflective writing

Confidentiality is a key ethical issue within health in terms of what is written and discussed (NMC, 2008). Patient confidentiality is prioritised, but corporate confidentiality is not always as easily considered. The Caldicott Committee has recommended that all items of information relating to an individual should be treated as potentially capable of identifying them and be appropriately protected to safeguard confidentiality (DH, 1997). Confidentiality means keeping information private. Corporate confidentiality means that institutions and organisations are also entitled to have their business kept private. This may be achieved by using a pseudonym and removing all identifiers that might locate the issues being written about. It is important when using someone else's information (such as a patient's case) to gain their consent for using the material for your learning.

There are concerns regarding the morality of using interpreted information about someone as a learning resource (Hargreaves, 1997). This applies to information about clients, or others, when writing reflectively, and creates an ethical dilemma. One method is to attempt to 'bracket' identifiers, thus focusing on the core issues. By stripping away all descriptors that cause distraction, the foundation issues are able to emerge and be decided upon. Johns' (2002) framework, as discussed in Chapter 4, offers an alternative by examining background philosophy, theory and problem presentation, as well as interpretation of reality, role and self-awareness in the form of questions, eliminating the necessity for descriptors. Philosophy relates to what kind of values and beliefs may be present in assumptions made about the problem, while theory is about the kind of framework that surrounds thinking about the problem. These will both be involved in how a problem is presented and in the interpretation of the reality of the problem. Questioning reflectively your own role and self-awareness in relation to the problem is necessary, and this seems a useful model to try.

Activity 9.2   *Reflection*

Using Johns' questions of philosophy, theory, problem presentation, interpretation of reality, role and self-awareness, write a reflective account of a recent episode relating to your practice.

As this activity relates to your practice, there is no outline answer at the end of the chapter.

Use of student and client knowledge needs to be ethically considerate, focusing on issues evaluatively and analytically, and examining personal parameters of responsibility. This applies to reflections on classroom discussions, group work or any other joint activity, which might be something that you intend to reflectively write about, regardless of whether or not you intend your writing to be seen by others. When others are not present to argue their case, or discuss issues with you in person, it is probably best to focus on issues rather than people. This means that others' confidentiality is assured and the professional role ethically protected (Brockbank and McGill, 1998). Read the following scenario and answer the questions at the end, to help you make sense of how you might approach these issues.

Scenario: Mia's reflection on collaborative learning

*Mia was a registered nurse who had trained overseas. She was working in a renal unit where two third-year nurses, Josh and Ray, were currently completing their placements. Mia had recently begun an Academic Development course, which taught her how to search for information and complete academic assignments, in order to prepare her for going on to study a mentorship programme. Mia was anxious because she was having difficulty in grasping the principles of reflection (something she was not used to as she had completed an exam-based course for her basic preparation). Mia had completed a formative piece of work reflecting on what she had learned on the programme so far, but the feedback from her tutor had indicated that she had failed substantially because she had not maintained confidentiality or reflected adequately. Mia was confused. She had identified the type of unit she worked in, as well as the **Trust** and where she was studying, but she had not named any of the patients. She had described her learning and what she wanted to do. Mia decided to ask Josh to help her, as he seemed to know a lot about reflection whenever she spoke about it at work. She was worried about '**losing face**' with her tutor.*

Mia asked Josh if he could explain how he reflected so that she could see what she was not doing. Josh asked Mia to think about her arrival in the Trust from the perspective of how she felt at the time and how she felt about it now. As Mia was describing this event from the different time perspectives, Josh asked her various questions, which he wrote down with her answers. At the end he asked Mia to read back what he had recorded from their dialogue. Mia was amazed at how Josh had captured her experience in a few words, but also how the questions had made her think differently about things. She decided to write about this process that evening and asked if Josh would look at it for her the next day.

Mia rewrote the piece of dialogue by including how she felt her knowledge had changed and how building relationships with people had made things easier. She was careful not to include Josh's name, but to relate the issue of developing knowledge through working and learning collaboratively with students. Mia did make some critical points about how her arrival could have been facilitated better.

Mia showed the piece she had written to Josh the next day. Josh made some helpful comments and identified a book that Mia might find helpful to inform her thinking about reflection. Mia felt more affirmed.

Questions

- In the scenario above, how did Mia breach confidentiality within her formative piece of writing?

continued . . .

- What might be the consequences for her and what might be the consequences for Josh if he breached confidentiality in a similar way in his written work?

There are outline answers to these questions at the end of the chapter.

Collaborative learning between those who are already qualified and students is a valuable process. This is especially useful when considering issues of confidentiality, to help the student understand the parameters of accountability and why qualified staff and mentors might see situations differently, or become anxious. Stripping away all descriptors could contribute to losing the context, therefore realistic description within consent might be a more reliable, as well as ethical, option. We proceed now to consider the role of personal reflective writing as a part of this process.

Personal reflective writing

Reflection in nursing has a dual function in supporting learning, but also supporting the individual. It requires considerable confidence to acknowledge limitations and deficits, and a degree of insight to admit these to oneself. According to Bolton (2010, p106), 'through the mirror' writing can make possible:

- leaps of understanding and connections;
- contact with unexamined thoughts and ideas;
- exploration of forgotten memories;
- expression and exploration of issues of which the writer is aware, but unable or unwilling otherwise to articulate.

From this perspective, such writing is always temporal and evolving, and may generate unexpected ideas. For example, when thinking about what caring means to you, you might suddenly remember when you were ill in bed at home as a child, and how wretched and unwell you felt. You might vividly *feel* the rumpled sheets and the resulting discomfort, the clamminess of the temperature, and how lonely you felt because all your friends were at school. This might make you revise more glib ideas of caring into something much more personal.

Making use of art forms such as poetry or scenes of a play may greatly increase the fluidity of expression and help deal with sometimes difficult emotions by helping these to take **cathartic** expression through the writing. Writing in this way develops a different articulation that can empower you, as the reader trying to make sense of your personal experience, to gain control of the emotions and issues involved in the reflection.

Richardson (1997) invites the reflective writer to find new forms of expression. To empower ourselves requires coming to know ourselves as being more than a professional identity. It is in knowing ourselves that we can hope to come to know our becoming too (Chan and Schwind, 2006). Poetic expression can express a unique part of who you are and does not necessarily have to follow any particular rules. It provides an opportunity for the playfulness described by Bolton (2010) at the outset as an essential part of going through the mirror, rather than becoming fixated with its surface. Poetry may not be something that everyone feels comfortable with, and it is not essential to use this form of expression, but try it out and you may surprise yourself. Remember, no one needs to see your writing. An example of poetry follows.

> What do you see when you look at me
>> A caring nurse or a man alone,
> What do you see when you look at me
>> A capable helper or someone losing his home,
> What do you see when you look at me
>> Someone missing class or trying to phone
> What do you see when you look at me
>> See the person, see the problem, see ME.

Undertaking the next activity will offer you the opportunity to express yourself differently.

Activity 9.3   *Reflection*

Think of something relating to your personal development that is very significant to you. Spend a little time reflecting on the situation or issue. Now try to write a reflection about it in the form of a poem or as scenes of a play. Reread this and consider what response and insights this form of expression elicits.

As this activity is based on your personal experiences, there is an outline answer to only part of this activity at the end of the chapter.

Personal writing may never be seen by another person, as it is a form of a diary that records your deepest impressions and considerations about what you are thinking and doing. This differs marginally from a reflective journal, which we proceed to consider next.

The reflective journal

While personal reflective writing can be cathartic and **catalytic**, helping you to let go of your emotions and achieve deep exploration (Driscoll, 2007), nevertheless there also needs to be reflection on how your role might develop as healthcare progresses. Logging reflective entries within a reflective journal helps to keep track of what you are learning and your practice experiences, including those you encounter through your preparation programme. In addition, such consistent writing helps to consider assessment, feedback and practice in terms of your whole experience, and thereby to integrate theory to practice.

As a nurse practitioner you are expected to keep a portfolio of evidence to demonstrate your learning for the regulatory body. At its simplest level, maintaining a reflective journal is a good starting point for demonstrating what and how you are learning. How you interact with different people is also important, as nursing is still about communicating with a variety of different people. Group dynamics are often key to the learning produced and warrant early attention (Jacques, 2000). Reflection and self-development play an increasing part in this process. Undertaking the next activity will help you to get started with logging such experience.

Activity 9.4   *Reflection*

Think of a recent experience (this could be from within the university or from practice). Now write about the following.

- Describe the experience.
- What essential factors contributed to this experience and are there significant features?

When you have kept your journal for a week or so, revisit it and consider the following.

- What are the themes emerging from the journal entries?
- What sense do you make of this and using what evidence?

As this activity is based on your personal experiences, there is an outline answer to only part of this activity at the end of the chapter.

Expressed dissatisfaction with others is a form of 'othering' that can remove responsibility and personal accountability for addressing the situation. When finding yourself starting to use 'othering', there is also the possibility, through reflection, to consciously reject following this route (Freshwater, 2000). Reflection and open dialogue are the best options to support trust in fragile circumstances, but could also be confronting for the less confident. Writing in your reflective journal how you intend to deal with the situation is a good starting point for taking proactive action, rather than leaving things to drift and relationships to suffer. The reflective journal is a useful tool for evaluating your strengths, interests and areas for development through reviewing such difficult issues and the emerging themes, as discussed at the start of the section. This review can inform your personal development planning, which is discussed next.

Personal development planning

Reflection creates vulnerability in terms of exposing thinking and practice to critique, and self-concept to realignment (Scanlan and Chernomas, 1997). This takes courage, cognitive insight and emotional fortitude. Planning involves reflecting on strengths and areas for improvement, and the interplay between the retrospective and prospective in shaping implementation strategies translating into concrete actions. Action that emanates from such processes requires daring and humility to try something new and to entertain the possibility of being wrong, as well as learning. This means making use of past learning experience to interpret present practice and knowledge when writing reflectively, and for personal development planning. This is an important point to consider when thinking about your learning contracts and whether they are product-, rather than process-focused.

A product-focused plan may be promoted by time constraints, but then arguably does not achieve the purpose, raising questions of accountability for both practice supervisors and learners. Feedback is an important component of reviewing progress, in that it provides evaluative information that can be reflected on and incorporated into planning future action and learning. It is important to have thought through what you are attempting to achieve, and potential commitment, in order to ensure that you can deliver consistently and equitably on undertakings you have given. It is important for clarity to articulate your own expectations when going into practice, or when being asked to complete independent study. Undertaking Activity 9.5 offers you an opportunity to think reflectively about these issues.

Activity 9.5   *Critical thinking*

Think about your next placement, or next year, if appropriate. If you are an experienced practitioner, think about your next appraisal. Now consider the following questions.

- What are your strengths?
- What are your weaknesses?
- How do you know this?
- What are you planning to do about this?
- What from reflection do you need to take forward?

Now write a reflective account to draw these parts into a whole as evidence for your portfolio.

As this activity is based on your personal experiences, there is an outline answer to only part of this activity at the end of the chapter.

Personal development planning is an important way to develop agency in your own learning and ensure that it is linked to your needs. In order to evidence your personal development you also need to write about it within formal assignments, whether you are a student on a preparation programme or an experienced practitioner undertaking study at university.

We proceed now to consider reflective writing in assignments.

Reflective writing in assignments

The professional voice is based on practice and 'knowing nursing' as an insider. The process nature of healthcare and educational practices makes this easier to articulate. In contrast, an academic voice in nursing is, seemingly, less certain, requiring intellectual effort to negotiate different viewpoints and parameters that are often erected. Reflection is a valuable part of the teaching and learning process, but needs to be purposeful and carefully constructed within curricula to achieve relevance and learning credibility. Threatening experiences may be buried and translated into more acceptable renditions to meet course, or curriculum, requirements or role achievement, rather than make sense of processes. For example, it may be difficult to write about mistakes for fear of punitive judgements. There is an ethical tension if issues do appear in reflective accounts from practice that appear unsound, or unsafe, as tutors may be professionally bound to do something while balancing confidentiality with a duty of care to the student. There needs to be clear outcomes for the process. Within this, both academic and practical ability can be shared more readily and thereby enable learning and build your confidence.

Marking of reflective writing in assignments is focused on the breadth and depth of the reflective content. This follows a continuum of whether written reflection and the conclusions reached are perceptive and significant with convincing conclusions, or whether reflection and its conclusions are superficial and lack relevance. Advancing to the further reaches of this continuum requires moving beyond description of reflection and offering perceptive reflection that ranges beyond the immediate context to include subtle thought and originality. This involves:

- considering what theoretical concepts are active in the situation;
- any unique features that the situation is demonstrating;
- what your view is, based on experience and reflection – give examples;
- keeping the focus on *your* practice and not generalising to some abstract generic view.

A brief example of a reflective paragraph that might be part of reflective writing in assignments is offered below.

Example of reflective writing in assignments

Having completed the complex healthcare module has made me think again about how I approach and think about people with complex illnesses. I realise that I am often focused on the task and forget about the patient experience. It can become easy to get caught up in problem solving and leave them out. Thinking only theoretically and cognitively separates me from important subjective and intuitive elements. It seems that, in this way, healthcare can become objectified rather than responding to the person. I need to communicate my decision making to the person better so that they can be included and be part of the solution. I will revisit person-centred care and decision-making literature and ensure that I include patients in my assessment and decision making in future. I will also discuss this with my mentor.

It sometimes helps to analyse reflection more deeply through guided reflection, as discussed in Chapter 8. When you are involved in guided reflection it is important to record the learning that this generates, in order to ensure that it is captured and not lost. We proceed to consider how this is another form of reflective writing.

Recording guided reflection

Guided reflection may also help address some of the ethical issues identified earlier of making students vulnerable, by providing support as well as clear outcomes for the process. The issue of a reconstructed past remains, although careful questioning of and attentive listening to oneself, as well as by the reflective guide, may highlight this. In order to record guided reflection, the following pro forma is offered, based on the one provided in Chapter 1.

PRO FORMA FOR DOCUMENTING GUIDED REFLECTION

Practice-based experience:

Main points identified from reflection on the experience:

Main points identified from guided exploration of the experience:

Learning points:

How will this learning be applied in practice?

Professional development achieved?

Chapter summary

Reflection too often dissolves in the reality of everyday work and life. Holism is achieved by embedding a continuous cycle of experimentation and review through reflective writing. Reflection is an art that requires insight and self-awareness, and it may take longer than the three years of a preparation programme, or continuing professional development programme, to develop fully. Writing is one way to start embedding the process. The activities in this chapter have provided different opportunities to expand your writing and develop different techniques that may generate further reflective insights.

Activities and scenarios: Brief outline answers

Activity 9.1: Reflection (page 120)

Maria is focused on how she is feeling and the impact on her learning. She has begun some superficial analysis of what Rachel could have done differently and what she might do to improve her remembering. Rachel considers both her own and Maria's feelings and the causes. She also analyses how her own actions have contributed to the current situation and what she can do about it. She plans actions for dealing with the stress she is feeling as well as ways of improving the atmosphere. Both Maria and Rachel have planned further action but neither has considered what consequences might result from their further actions. Analysing these further could add depth to the reflection, as could considering the actions and influence of others and how events can influence future behaviour.

Activity 9.3: Reflection (page 125)

While the content and structure of your reflection is likely to be unique to you, there are some common rules you might have followed. You might have plotted the reflective story as a sequence of scenes. If using poetic devices, you might have considered whether to use a chorus or rhyming mechanisms to emphasise particular points. All of these considerations are important.

Activity 9.4: Reflection (page 126)

The themes you identified might have been concerned with communication skills, decision making and relationships with peers, practice colleagues, clients and tutors.

Activity 9.5: Critical thinking (page 127)

You might have identified strengths in relation to particular skills and others that you wanted to improve. It is possible that confidence could also have featured as an area for improvement. How you would know this would be from feedback from others and your own reflections. What you intend to do about the areas identified is probably learn more, which for the experienced practitioner might involve some kind of study day or training as well. If you are a student, this should inform your writing of your learning contract. Your reflection following planning your personal development is likely to be much more positive, as you have developed some agency in your learning and development. (For the discussion on agency, return to Chapter 3.)

Scenario: Faheed's experience of group cultural differences (page 121)

Faheed might have learned how sharing his experience with the group has helped to inspire them and given him confidence. He might also have learned more about his communication and assertiveness skills. He might have identified that he can lead others. He might also have identified how to break down barriers between different professions.

Scenario: Mia's reflection on collaborative learning (pages 123–4)

Mia broke corporate confidentiality by naming the healthcare Trust that she worked in and the institution where she was studying. This meant that her work could, potentially, identify where any situation she was talking about was located. Some people call this the 'on the bus test'. Should the work be left in a public place, are there sufficient identifiers to locate where situations are happening? In terms of the consequences of breaching confidentiality, for Mia these would be greater (although these are still dependent on the seriousness of the breach), because she is a registered nurse and therefore accountable for her actions. The consequences for Josh, as a student, if he had followed the same actions as Mia, are less serious (although these are still dependent on the seriousness of the breach), because he has a responsibility for maintaining confidentiality but is not yet a registered accountable practitioner. The best option is to leave any identifiers out of any account!

Further reading

Bolton, G (2010) *Reflective Practice: Writing and professional development*. Los Angeles, CA: Sage.

This book offers an in-depth guide to reflective writing, which is beyond the scope of this chapter.

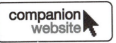

For further activities and other useful material, visit the companion website at **www.sagepub.co.uk/howatson-jones_reflective2e**

Chapter 10
Using new media for reflecting

continued . . .

By the second progression point:

6.   Forms appropriate and constructive professional relationships with families and other carers.

Cluster: Organisational aspects of care

12.   People can trust the newly registered graduate nurse to respond to their feedback and a wide range of other sources to learn, develop and improve services.

By the first progression point:

1.   Works within *The Code* (NMC, 2008) and adheres to the *Guidance on Professional Conduct for Nursing and Midwifery Students* (NMC, 2010b).

By the second progression point:

4.   Reflects on own practice and discusses issues with other members of the team to enhance learning.

Chapter aims

After reading this chapter, you will be able to:

*   identify different types of new media that can be used for reflection;
*   assess the advantages and avoid the pitfalls of using new media for reflection;
*   develop a reflective script for a new media narrative;
*   identify how you can contribute to others' reflective learning.

Case study: Sonia's reflective wiki experience

Sonia has just started her child nursing preparation programme. One of the first tasks she is asked to do is to set up a wiki with different pages for different parts of her learning experience. Sonia is a bit concerned about completing this task because she has never used a wiki before. However, after an introductory talk about how to get started from her course tutor, Julie, Sonia is able to set up her personal wiki with named pages for graduate skills, reflective diary, IT skills, practice and professional development. Sonia shares her wiki with Julie so that she can get feedback on her writing.

Sonia starts to use her reflective diary page to log her learning experiences of lectures. She mentions her clinical science tutor by name, saying how impressed she is with the resources he provides to the class. Julie places a comment on the page that confidentiality needs to be maintained by not including people's names. Sonia goes back to the wiki page and edits out the clinical science tutor's name.

When Sonia starts her first placement she is very excited. She decides that it would be helpful for her learning to reflect on these early experiences. Each week she writes a reflective log about what she has learned in placement.

continued . . .

> *Remembering Julie's comment about maintaining confidentiality, Sonia ensures that she does not name any people, the placement or the organisation where it is located. Julie places a further comment on Sonia's practice wiki page affirming Sonia's reflective ability and her progression and learning from the feedback that she receives.*

Introduction

As technology progresses rapidly new media are constantly becoming available. This means that different opportunities for creative ways of reflecting are increasing. It is important in the digital age to become familiar with the diverse range of options available not only to ensure that you make use of what is available, but also so that you are able to engage with and teach others. However, as highlighted in the case study, new media also pose some potential problems that you need to guard against in order to protect those in your care and avoid misconduct resulting from not adhering to *The Code*.

This chapter will introduce some of the new media that you might use in your reflective learning. It will also highlight the opportunities and dangers posed by such media and identify ways that you can use new media responsibly and professionally. The chapter will also offer you an opportunity to develop a reflective script. The chapter will conclude with how to translate this into a digital story.

Different types of new media

New media refers to new technological tools that have become available in recent years and that make connecting through the worldwide web much easier. Some of these new technological tools are:

- social networking;
- instant messaging;
- tweets;
- Skype;
- e-mail;
- texting;
- creative digital media.

Ohler (2008) uses the term 'new media' because it allows for expansion and change in an evolving medium. New media offer different possibilities for reflection. As has already been highlighted in the case study at the start of this chapter, wikis offer structure as well as the opportunity for feedback when they are shared. Because the wiki is like an electronic filing cabinet where information can be stored under subject headings, it is useful for keeping a reflective log. It can either be kept private within the virtual learning environment or shared with others who have to be invited by you and accept the link you send them. Feedback is given via a comments button.

Virtual learning environments can also include e-portfolio tools where you can log experiences and information for building your portfolio. Your portfolio should include a section of reflective learning as this is a key aspect of the nursing code of conduct in terms of keeping your knowledge up to date (NMC, 2008). The NMC expects all nurses to keep a portfolio and can call on this evidence at the point of registration and beyond (see *Successful Professional Portfolios for Nursing Students* (Reed, 2011), in this series).

Social networking is useful for sharing ideas. It enables discussion of issues, sharing learning and following key experts through blogs. However, open sites such as Facebook and Twitter need to be used with caution, as will be discussed later in this chapter.

Creative media allow you to upload images and audio to create digital stories offering the potential for more creative reflection. Examples of free downloadable media programs that enable you to do this include Photo Story 3, Audacity and Windows Movie Maker. These can be used to create media files from the images, sounds and narration that you input. This harnesses different thought processes. For example, you might choose an image as a metaphor for what would require many words to explain. The viewer makes sense of the meaning framed by his or her own biographical experience (for more information on this, revisit Chapter 3). Creating stories requires discipline, structure, scripting, critical analysis and editing, which are also the skills needed for critical reflection. Complete the activity below to consider how you might use new media.

Activity 10.1   *Reflection*

- In what ways do you think you might use the different media mentioned to reflect?
- Are there any other media not mentioned that you could use?

As this activity is based on your experience, there is no outline answer at the end of the chapter.

You might have considered how different forms of media allow you to interact with others to get feedback on your ideas and to develop your reflective thinking and experience. However, while interaction can be an advantage, there are also some pitfalls to beware of. These are discussed in more detail in the next section.

Advantages and pitfalls of new media

New media, as has already been suggested, enable dynamic articulation of reflections. This includes synchronous approaches such as social networking as well as asynchronous methods such as discussion boards and blogs. The advantages of these are that they bring nurses together in new ways, providing opportunities for development, for making nurses' voices heard and for sharing good practice (Falconer, 2011). For example, through talking to nurses from other countries it is possible to compare and contrast different healthcare systems across the world and reflect upon your own role at the same time. New media also make it easier to study at a distance and to keep in contact with developing ideas without having to sit in a classroom with others. This makes education programmes more accessible to a wider variety of people.

However, there are also inherent risks. In a recent discussion at the Royal College of Nursing (RCN) (2011) congress, David Jones highlighted that once information has been shared on a website it cannot be removed. Recognising that nurses use social networking sites, the NMC (2012) has produced some guidance, noting that nurses and midwives will put their registration at risk and students may jeopardise their ability to join the register if they:

- share confidential information online;
- post inappropriate comments about staff or patients;
- use social networking sites to bully and intimidate colleagues;
- pursue personal relationships with patients and service users;
- distribute sexually explicit material;
- use social networking sites in a way that is unlawful.

The NMC advises that conduct in the real world and online should be viewed as one and the same, and conduct should always be in keeping with the standards of *The Code* (NMC, 2008). The RCN (2009) has also produced legal advice on using the internet. This emphasises the importance of reading and adhering to the IT policy of the organisation you are in and ensuring that you uphold the reputation of both your profession and the organisation. For the student nurse this would mean the organisations within which your preparation programme and your placements are located. The RCN (2009, p2) recommends that you:

- *avoid any identification of your employer;*
- *under no circumstances identify patients in your care or post information that might lead to the identification of a patient;*
- *do not air grievances where others might read them;*
- *do not make disparaging remarks about an employer, colleagues or clients.*

Most of this is straightforward advice to follow, but there are times when boundaries blur and it can be difficult to remember who you are professionally. Consider the following case study and complete Activity 10.2 to clarify what you think you would do.

Case study: Alistair's social networking experience

Alistair was working in the community on placement with practice nurses at a GP surgery. He enjoyed this placement because of the diversity of the work and the people he came into contact with. He became very friendly with his mentor, Colin. Alistair asked Colin if he would be interested in becoming a friend on his social networking site. Colin agreed and told Alistair to send him an invitation. That evening Alistair was on the site and sent Colin an invitation to become a friend. In his invitation Alistair said that he very much enjoyed working with Colin at the GP surgery. Colin accepted the invitation and he and Alistair have been swapping messages about their interests outside work. There are some issues that Alistair wants to learn more about in relation to his placement, but he does not discuss these on the social networking site because this would not be appropriate. He catches up with Colin at work about them instead. At the end of his placement Alistair asks Colin to keep in touch, which he agrees to do.

Activity 10.2   *Critical thinking*

After reading the above case study, answer the following questions.

- What are the main issues in this case study?
- What might be the outcomes for Alistair and Colin?
- What might you do differently?

There are outline answers to these questions at the end of the chapter.

The above activity has offered you the opportunity to think about some of the difficulties involved in separating professional and private life and keeping to appropriate boundaries, particularly when you feel that people are friends. Reflecting on such experiences is important for developing and maintaining professional behaviour. Your professional integrity is essential to becoming registered or keeping your registration if you are a registered practitioner. We proceed to consider positive ways in which new media can be used for reflection by exploring how to develop stories.

Developing a reflective story using new media

Storytelling has been a traditional part of human communication for centuries and stories are a useful pedagogical tool for developing understanding (Abrahamson, 1998). Considering a significant issue and creating the story that surrounds it helps to clarify your thinking and reasoning and to reflect differently than is possible in a written assignment (Matthews-DeNatale, 2008). According to Boase (2008, p9), developing reflective stories using new media enables you to:

- *promote deep reflection, review, analysis and ordering of information (e.g. a project, a topic, an experience);*
- *value emotional/personal input;*

- *make sense of experience;*
- *encourage cooperative activity;*
- *create powerful end products that can have a transformative effect on maker and viewer alike;*
- *develop capacity for self-review;*
- *build confidence.*

The process of creating the story helps to make it an embodied experience, which is so important for deepening your understanding and learning. What is meant by embodiment is that the experience is lived and owned by you as the person reflecting, and unconscious aspects are brought to light. Our experiences are informed by the *appearance, disappearance and reappearance of events and people making our world seem familiar* (Horsdal, 2012, p10). However, we cannot perceive these influences unless we are able to see the whole story. To do this you need first to develop a script, an example of which can be seen below.

A script about person-centred care

'Where's Mike?,' asked the menacing-looking individual at the desk. Maggie glanced at me nervously. 'Room 9,' I calmly replied. He walked up the corridor and disappeared into Mike's room. Mike had been transferred to the limb surgery unit following a motorcycle accident. He had been filtering to go off a roundabout and had been crushed by a lorry. His lower leg was damaged beyond repair and had to be amputated. Mike was struggling to come to terms with his injury, often becoming angry and resentful. The man visiting him was clearly a motorcyclist too.

This is my first qualified nurse post and I am still getting used to it. I am learning how to dress stump wounds and bandage them correctly. What I am finding harder, though, is learning how to connect with the wounded person. I come from a background where people are valued as individuals and I want to use those values in my nursing. The problem is, how do I work with Mike in a way that is meaningful for him and that values his individuality?

We start to chat. Mike says that he finds the Limb Surgery Unit boring because there is nothing for him to do. I ask him what he normally does. He says that he works on art designs for motorcycles. He has a website where he showcases his work and people contact him or they approach him at the events he attends. He doesn't want to miss the motorcycle show at the end of the month. He is worried that his business will suffer. I talk to the occupational therapist and ask her to source some art materials for Mike. Mike starts to use these to create design ideas and appears more purposeful. I also talk to the physiotherapist about his objective of getting to the motorcycle show. The physiotherapist tailors Mike's exercise regime to include walking on uneven terrain.

At the end of the month Mike's friend, who no longer appears to be menacing as we have come to know him better, takes Mike to the motorcycle show. I think I will ask Mike if he is willing to share his experiences and recovery with others as we do get a number of biker patients.

Read the following case study and then complete Activity 10.3.

Case study: Naeve's critical incident experience

Naeve was working in a mental health secure unit placement. She was in the third year of her mental health nurse preparation programme and due to finish in three months. She had just finished a stretch of duties and on one of her days off decided to reflect on a particular issue that had given her work satisfaction. The unit had some patients with complex problems. One of these was Jeff, who had been sectioned and admitted after smashing up the family home and a stand-off with police. He had been off work with severe stress preceding this event. His family had found the experience of his outburst extremely traumatic and were reluctant to visit him. He had a sister who lived two hours' travelling time away. Naeve could see that Jeff was withdrawn and did not speak much. Each day that she was on shift she spent some time sitting with him, trying to draw him out. By the second week he was starting to mumble some responses. By the third week Naeve managed to coax Jeff to come downstairs for his lunch. His sister had been enquiring after Jeff regularly. In that third week Naeve asked Jeff if he wanted to see his sister and he agreed. Jeff asked for Naeve to be present when they met.

Jeff's sister Miriam met him in the common room. At first everything appeared to be going well, but then Jeff lost his temper when Miriam asked him where he would go on leaving the unit because he could not go back home. Naeve ushered Miriam out of the room and returned to Jeff. Although she felt anxious inside, Naeve was able to maintain a calm exterior which gradually helped Jeff to calm down. Naeve's mentor, Andrew, had been observing her communication interactions over this period of time and was very impressed with Naeve's handling of this volatile situation. Andrew gave Naeve a glowing report prior to her leaving this placement.

Naeve used new media in the form of a private blog to reflect on the incident and her overall feelings about the placement over the last few weeks. She felt she had made some real progress in her communication and interaction with Jeff. She found this satisfying as it appeared to affirm her communication ability. When Jeff had become agitated and angry in his interaction with his sister, Naeve had reacted quickly to remove Miriam from danger and calm the situation despite feeling a bit fearful herself. She knew that this was part of what she would need to do as a mental health nurse and was pleased that the way she had handled the critical incident had been affirmed by her mentor, Andrew. When she considered what she might have done differently she thought about whether she should have called for help, or sent Miriam to get help when she left the room. The reason she had not done this was because she felt confident in her own abilities and the therapeutic relationship she had established with Jeff. Naeve thought that the worst that could have happened was that Jeff might have struck her, but as she had had training in breakaway techniques she felt able to take care of herself to get away if necessary, but she preferred to use communication to resolve the situation. The incident had increased her confidence in being able to manage different situations effectively and she felt more prepared for qualifying in the next few months.

Activity 10.3   *Critical thinking*

Use the case study above to develop a story script about the incident and Naeve's reflection on it.

There is an outline answer to this activity at the end of the chapter.

If you want to have another go, write a story script for a critical incident you have experienced and your reflection on it.

As this activity is based on your experience, there is no answer at the end of the chapter.

Writing an event as a script helps you to deconstruct and examine different elements before reassembling them in a cohesive whole. A script normally starts with a significant event. As such, the script grabs the reader's attention at the start and has an unfolding plot that connects different aspects in a whole (Boase, 2008). This requires critical awareness in knowing what to select and what to leave out and how to substantiate important points. The script should be approximately 200–300 words in length (Matthews-DeNatale, 2008). As stated by Boase (2008, p10), the skills involved in creating a story using new media include:

- *narrative generation;*
- *reflection;*
- *analysis of material;*
- *analysis of self in relation to material;*
- *organising and sorting information for use;*
- *use of personal and technological/technical skills.*

The next step is to convert the script into an audio file using an appropriate audio editing tool. An example is Audacity, which records you narrating the script. Try to do this in as natural a way as possible in a quiet space, as if you were talking to someone. This is the first step to converting the script into a digital story. The next step is to match the script with appropriate images. To do this you will need to access the software that you intend to use and create a storyboard, which allows you to place your chosen images on an editing line similar to a film strip. Images can be sourced from your own photographs, from photo-share sites such as www.flickr.com and from hand drawings. It is important to make sure that you check and follow copyright rules for any shared images and that you gain consent for any personal photos involving other people. Once you have matched your audio with the images you can add titles and save your project. At this stage you should still be able to edit it. You are now ready to review your project file and reflect on whether the story portrays what you intended. It is also helpful at this stage to get other people's feedback because then you can make editing changes before completing the final story package. Complete Activity 10.4 to see what you can produce.

Activity 10.4   *Reflection*

(Note: You will need a headset with a microphone for this activity.)

Download Photo Story 3 from http://microsoft-photo-story.en.softonic.com/ on to your computer.

- Find a photo that holds special meaning for you.
- Think about the memories that are triggered by the photo and write a story script about these using the guidance previously given.
- Translate this script into a digital story using the new media software and following the prompts, as suggested above.
- Review your digital story and the processes used to create it and reflect on what you have learned.

As this activity is based on your own experiences, there is no outline answer at the end of the chapter.

We proceed now to explore how sharing stories that have been created using new media can contribute to the reflective learning of others.

Contributing to the reflective learning of others

Sharing your development of the digital story with peers and teachers not only helps you to increase the quality of the final product, but also contributes to the reflective learning of others as they explore the meaning that they make from viewing your story. It is therefore useful to share your practice with others in order to collaborate in reflecting. As technology progresses new media are increasingly being used within nurse preparation programmes to bring the service-user voice to the fore and to develop learning in more engaging ways. Examples that are used can be found on the Patient Voices website at www.patient-voices.org. It is interesting to view different stories and to share your reflections on them.

Chapter summary

This chapter has explored how to use new media to develop reflection in different ways. Some of the advantages and pitfalls have been highlighted to help you use these new opportunities constructively and guard against creating problems for yourself that could affect you professionally and jeopardise your registration. The activities have offered you opportunities to develop your own digital story to reflect upon. In the process you will have developed new media skills that you can take forward in your own learning and can use to contribute to the reflections of others.

Activities and scenarios: Brief outline answers

Activity 10.2 Critical thinking (page 137)

The main issues that arise in this case study are:

- the blurring of Alistair's and Colin's professional and private lives as evidenced in their social networking communication;
- Alistair's mention in his invitation that they both work in a GP surgery.

The potential outcomes for Alistair are that, because Colin is his mentor, any feedback that Colin gives him may be viewed by Alistair through the lens of their social networking communications rather than in a professional light. Alistair's professional behaviour could therefore be affected. The potential outcomes for Colin are that he is accountable for his actions and could be putting his registration at risk. By blurring the boundary between his professional role as Alistair's mentor and communicating socially with him online, he cannot be sure what Alistair might say that other people could see and that could have professional repercussions for him. If you were the student in this situation you might think that it was not appropriate to develop a friendship with someone in a position to decide your future. If you were the qualified mentor you might think it was not appropriate to develop a friendship with someone whose future you are deciding. You might also think about the potential risk to your registration of social networking with someone while you are also mentoring them in a professional capacity. Reflecting on this you might decide that both of you need to inform yourselves about policies and guidance on using new media within your organisations and from a regulation perspective.

Activity 10.3: Critical thinking (page 140)

The script might go as follows:

'Get out you stupid woman,' he shouted, raising his fist at his sister. I hurriedly ushered her out of the room and then went back to try to calm him down. He had come to the unit after smashing up his home and threatening the police and his family. For the last three weeks I have been trying to build up a therapeutic relationship with him to get him to communicate and come out of himself more. I had not intended for him to react like this, though, when I told his sister he was ready to see her. I should be scared, but I feel calm. He is out of control, but I feel in control of the situation. The preparation I have had has, I think, helped me to feel this way. What would I do if he hits me? Others might say 'It is your own fault because you did not ask for help.' I would have to rethink my strategy. But for now things are calming down. I go home feeling great after the glowing report from my mentor. My communication strategies have been rewarded and affirmed by the patient calming down and my mentor praising my handling of the situation. I feel ready to progress towards being a qualified nurse.

Further reading

Nursing and Midwifery Council (NMC) (2012) *Social Networking Sites.* Available online at www.nmc-uk.org/Nurses-and-midwives/Advice-by-topic/A/Advice/Social-networking-sites.

Reed, S (2011) *Successful Professional Portfolios for Nursing Students.* Exeter: Learning Matters.

Royal College of Nursing (RCN) (2009) *Legal Advice for RCN Members Using the Internet.* London: RCN. Available online at www.rcn.org.uk/__data/assets/pdf_file/0008/272195/003557.pdf.

Useful websites

http://digitalstorytelling.coe.uh.edu This website offers a tutorial and a range of guidance on creating your own digital story.

http://digitalstorytelling.coe.uh.edu/personal_reflection.html This website offers examples of a variety of reflective digital stories that can be viewed using different media.

www.nmc-uk.org This website provides information on the latest regulations and what nurses and midwives need to do to adhere to them.

www.patient-voices.org This website offers a range of stories involving patients and nurses in diverse settings and situations. These provide useful examples for this genre of storytelling.

www.rcn.org.uk This website offers advice and guidance on issues relating to nursing. It also has discussion forums where nurses can share practice.

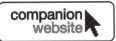

For further activities and other useful material, visit the companion website at **www.sagepub.co.uk/howatson-jones_reflective2e**

Chapter 11
Critical reflection

continued . . .

8. People can trust the newly registered graduate nurse to gain their consent based on sound understanding and informed choice prior to any intervention and that their rights in decision making and consent will be respected and upheld.

By the first progression point:

1. Seeks consent prior to sharing confidential information outside of the professional care team, subject to agreed safeguarding and protection procedures.

Cluster: Organisational aspects of care

15. People can trust the newly registered graduate nurse to safely delegate to others and to respond appropriately when a task is delegated to them.

By the first progression point:

1. Accepts delegated activities within limitations of own role, knowledge and skill.

Chapter aims

After reading this chapter you will be able to:

- critically examine personal contributions and those of others within practical and psychological considerations;
- explore the limits of your understanding;
- assess sources of evidence within any situation;
- identify the coming together of new ideas.

Example story

Meg was in the third year of her nurse preparation programme. On her way home from an early shift, she stopped at the supermarket. As Meg rounded the corner to the dairy aisle, she came across a man on the floor. Meg placed him in the recovery position and observed that he appeared stiff and rigid and was **cyanosed**. Meg recognised this as the **tonic** phase of an **epileptic fit** and cleared a space around him so that, as the **clonic** phase of jerking started, he would not injure himself. Meg continued to monitor that he started breathing again as the tonic phase gave way to the clonic phase. At this point someone came up to Meg and told her he was a first aider and that she should put something between the man's teeth to stop him biting his tongue. Meg was not sure whether this was right and decided not to follow the advice. The store staff had called an ambulance and, when the paramedics arrived, Meg told them what she had done and then completed her shopping and went home.

When she got home Meg was surprised to find she was rather shaken by the event. She tried to analyse what had happened and why she was feeling this way. She realised that her shakiness was a reaction to the adrenaline rush she had experienced on finding the man collapsed on the floor. While this had helped to focus her mind on what was important, it also had the physiological consequences that she was now experiencing.

Meg critically reflected upon her actions. Looking back, she thought that perhaps she should have checked the man for other signs, such as looking at his pupils and checking for any injury, as there are a number of reasons why someone might be fitting. She was satisfied to have put the man in the recovery position so quickly and to have protected his airway. Meg thought about what the person claiming to be a first aider had said about putting something between the man's teeth. As she still was not sure, she decided to check what her nursing literature recommended and found that this action was positively discouraged. Meg was glad she had not listened, but also thought critically about what had led her to this decision. Turning someone into the recovery position was a way to ensure the tongue did not fall back and block the airway, and therefore pushing something into the mouth at the same time was likely to achieve the opposite effect and potentially force the tongue backwards. Meg had instinctively grasped the danger and avoided it. However, she realised that, had she been in the first year of her preparation programme, she might have listened, assuming that the man claiming to be a first aider was correct. This led her to reflect on how anyone can know the experience, qualifications and knowledge of anyone who stops to help in an emergency. It was really important in such situations to work within her own competence and knowledge levels so as not to do harm. Meg was glad that she had waited for the ambulance staff to help instead. She decided that she would do a more thorough initial assessment in future to ensure that she did not miss anything important.

Introduction

Part of becoming a professional is about developing criticality in order to identify, through analysis, what are significant priorities and potential solutions. As you progress through your preparation programme you will be able to develop critical skills from first observations to more complex decision making.

This chapter emphasises the intense nature of critical reflection and its relevance to the developing skill of criticality. It will also offer you opportunities to engage in critical reflection through different activities and scenarios. How new ideas come together as the final part of an analytical process will be considered at the end.

Critically examining personal contributions and those of others

Critical reflection differs from other forms of reflection in that it examines and questions all the factors involved in a situation from a critical perspective, which makes the familiar unfamiliar. This means looking at routine situations as if they were new in order to find out what might be seen differently. This requires disciplined thought to achieve the depth of analysis required. Such a questioning approach is also directed at personal actions in order to investigate motives, assumptions and decision making, and what you were really thinking. The frameworks offered in Chapter 4 provide encompassing structures that can be used to direct and complete such a critical approach. Combining this with critical incident analysis, such as reviewing and analysing situations that are important for learning, can help to build case studies from which to learn (Rolfe, 2011). Undertaking Activity 11.1 can help you to begin critical incident analysis and develop your learning by examining your own contributions and those of others within situations in order to learn from them.

Activity 11.1   *Critical thinking*

Critical incident analysis is a form of debrief that looks back at situations in order to consider what might need to be learned. Review what you have done, or been involved with, in the last few weeks and choose an incident to review. Write a detailed account of the event, including your own and others' actions. Now consider the following questions.

- Why is this situation significant for you?
- How did it affect you?
- How did you feel about it?
- What was satisfying about the situation?
- What was concerning about the situation?
- What might you have done differently?
- Was there any additional knowledge that you needed?
- What have you learned?
- How will you take this learning forward?

There are outline answers to this activity at the end of the chapter.

Having reviewed your incident, you might like to go further by considering who was responsible and who was accountable in the situation, and any implications in terms of significance, concerns and potential consequences. How does this inform your thinking about being a nurse?

As this is based on your own experiences, there is no outline answer at the end of the chapter.

Examining situations in this systematic way may be time-consuming but ensures that situations and cases are *studied* for what can be learned and what can be taken forward with situational and experiential evidence. Connecting this with other forms of knowledge helps to add to the evidence base. Critical incident analysis may be undertaken with positive or negative situations. Consider the following case study to see how this might be done.

Case study: Elimu's compliment

Elimu was in the final year of his nurse preparation programme and working on a stroke unit. This was an extended placement, enabling Elimu to really get to know the patients and staff and feel a part of the team. Elimu was putting into practice the management principles that he was learning on his nurse preparation programme. During a particularly busy shift, one of the patients suffered a cardiac arrest. Elimu was close by and called for help and then calmly initiated the resuscitation protocol. At the end of the shift his mentor complimented Elimu on his swift actions, calm manner and correct responses.

Elimu thought about this critically on his way home, deconstructing the chain of events and reviewing his actions. He considered whether there had been any warning signs that perhaps he might have missed that the patient was about to arrest, but the nursing observations he had recorded earlier had not changed. Elimu felt that he had responded as quickly as was possible and his response was linked to good visual observation of his patients. He had called for help so that the resuscitation team could be alerted and other staff would join him. This had resulted in someone bringing the necessary equipment. In the meantime, Elimu had been able to commence cardiopulmonary resuscitation because he had learnt how to do this in class. He analysed how this felt different from practising on the simulation dummy. He needed to concentrate on the amount of force he used in order to maintain consistency. It was also much more tiring than he had anticipated, confirming another reason to seek help.

As part of his management course Elimu had discussed different types of leadership and delegation in a variety of situations, and this knowledge helped him to respond calmly and effectively. However, Elimu recognised that his knowledge of the different drugs that the team used when they arrived was limited. He decided that learning these was something he would take forward from the situation. However, his mentor's compliment had affirmed his actions and so he recognised that these were appropriate to the situation.

The case study identifies the importance of the team for responding to situations and for peer feedback. Interpersonal relationships are an important source of team building and peer support, and are fertile ground for critically examining personal contributions and those of others. Anyone new to practice, including the student nurse, relies on peers when entering new environments (Petty, 2009). Peer support also involves being able to offer constructive feedback in order to develop practice. This can be hard to do as it is easy to become critical rather than critically constructive about personal contributions and those of others.

Trust is an issue that needs to be developed in order to facilitate learning critically. Building trust involves three arenas comprising risk, example and consistency (Curzon-Hobson, 2002). Reflection and open dialogue are helpful to support trust in fragile circumstances. Students can find integrating into an unknown environment with its own established team quite intimidating, whether this is a programme, a new module, or a new placement area in practice (Dix and Hughes, 2004). Consider the following scenario to reflect critically on integrating new members of staff into a team.

Scenario: Integrating a new member of staff

A new member of staff recently joined the team. The new member of staff requires constant attention and support, making it difficult for me to get on with my job. I have allocated time to catch up, but she still constantly interrupts me for guidance, instead of problem solving for herself. She is also given exceptional leeway as to flexi working time to accommodate her childcare, which is now putting extra pressure on the rest of us as we have to manage after she has gone early.

Questions
- After critically reflecting on this scenario, what do you think are the main points from the perspectives of both the experienced practitioner and the new member of staff?
- What potential learning points have you identified and how might these be applied in practice?

There are outline answers to these questions at the end of the chapter.

Being able to critically examine personal contributions in relationship with others also, potentially, opens up a different point of view that is more empathic and therefore supportive of staff relations. This leads to more positive atmospheres, where it is possible to offer constructive critique from which people do not take offence, but from which they learn the limits of their understanding. We proceed to explore how critical reflection can help to address limits in understanding in the next section.

Exploring the limits of understanding

Critically reflecting on the limits of your understanding is of prime importance for the novice and experienced practitioner and is enshrined within the code of conduct (NMC, 2008). Even if you have previously been competent in a skill or developed understanding of certain knowledge, both of these can decay over time. Equally, healthcare is also constantly evolving so that things change and new learning is required. Therefore, by maintaining a critically reflective stance to your practice you will be able to perceive deficits in your knowledge and skills base, and the limits of your understanding. Writing reflections in a journal facilitates analysing experience, creating new ideas and awareness of new learning (Chirema, 2007). To do this involves critically reviewing daily experience and analysing it, raising awareness of how you are learning and what new knowledge you are developing. From Tappen et al.'s (2004, p287) perspective, critical thinking requires individuals to:

- impose the criteria of reasoning, such as precision, relevance, depth and accuracy;
- become aware of all assumptions and points of view in an argument;
- continually assess the process of thinking;
- determine strengths, limitations and implications of the thinking.

For example, when thinking about why you react in particular ways to certain situations, you may impose a psychological reasoning process and compare your responses to those set within the criteria. You may then question the assumptions you have used and assess your thinking in relation to these. Determining strengths, limitations and implications involves imagining the possible consequences of thinking in this way. Consider the case study to identify how thinking critically can be a starting point for critical reflection.

Case study: Rob's dyslexia

Rob was in the first year of his nurse preparation programme. He had not had an easy time in learning at school, and he was finding the programme was becoming harder now that he had to complete several written assignments. Rob decided to reflect critically on the problems with his learning and explore the options available to him.

Rob considered the problems he had with reading and writing, and how he would never have an easy time in formal learning. He realised that he was never going to be able to retain information in the same way that others could when he related his abilities to the graduate skills that were expected of him. Although Rob considered that he was good at creative problem solving and working with people, he was also concerned that he would never be able to function at the same level as other practitioners did. Rob realised that, in order to move forward, he had to first overcome his fear.

When reflecting critically, Rob realised that the way that he saw things differently was actually a positive thing in that he could see alternative solutions that others could not. But Rob also perceived that he needed structure to help him understand what to do when learning new concepts, and this was why he found self-directed study and activities hard. Rob noted that he tended to write himself notes and scribble as a way of reinforcing particular points. Handouts did not help him as he tended to focus more on people talking.

Rob spoke to the study support department at his university. He also asked his tutors whether he could audio-record their teaching. Using this strategy meant that he could write down what was important when listening in class and when listening to the recording later. In this way he was able to access the information better. This gave him more idea of what to write about in his assignments as well as a chance to be reflective.

The case study may have helped you to identify that limits to understanding may also relate to ability to engage with study. This is an important area to critique in order for you to be able to reflectively find strategies that work for you. Undertaking Activity 11.2 can help you to identify limits to your understanding and ways to address these.

Activity 11.2 — *Reflection*

Think about a recent situation where you were not sure what to do. Consider the following questions.

- What alerted you to the uncertainty?
- What did you know?
- What did you not know?
- What were the consequences?
- What might have been the consequences if you had known?
- What can you do about this?
- What learning do you take from this situation?

As this activity is based on your own experiences, there is no outline answer at the end of the chapter.

You may have identified that there are specific areas you need to learn more about, or that there are some skills that you need to develop. This is part of being a reflective practitioner and important to continue. Consider the following scenario of how exploring limits to knowledge can also be an important safety issue.

Scenario: Fajid's understanding of young carers

Fajid was in the first year of his children's nurse preparation programme. He was on his third placement, which was with the school nurses. His mentor, Simon, involved Fajid in **health promotion** activities, working with schools on their healthy eating strategies. He was also involved in vaccination sessions. Part of the school nurse role was to support pupils who had behavioural problems and follow up absenteeism. Simon was currently working with Kate who was a young carer for her mum. Simon and Fajid visited her at home to assess the situation and find ways to empower Kate. Fajid discussed Kate's situation when he and Simon left the house. He wondered why Kate, who was only 14 years old, was left caring for her mother.

Question
- What are the limits to Fajid's understanding in this scenario? What might be the consequences for Kate, her mum and Fajid?

There is an outline answer to this question at the end of the chapter.

In the above scenario Simon could help Fajid's learning by asking him to reflect critically on his actions and the potential consequences, in a similar way to what the question is asking you to do. Identifying the sources of evidence used and rectifying deficits are important to maintaining safe practice. In the next section, we proceed to critically assessing the sources of evidence in a given situation.

Assessing sources of evidence within the situation

There is a need for novice and experienced practitioners to reflect critically on the evidence base of their actions in order to provide good-quality patient care and identify their learning needs. This means examining the sources of evidence used when planning patient care and making decisions. You may be a novice or an experienced practitioner, but critically examining the evidence used within the situations you find yourself in is an important part of developing your practice at any stage. Undertaking Activity 11.3 can help you to consider the sources of evidence used in a situation from your experience.

Activity 11.3   *Critical thinking*

Think of a situation from your experience in practice. Examine the sources of evidence supporting your interpretations and your decision making, using the following questions.

- How did you assess the situation?
- What was your assessment based on?
- How did you know what to base it on?
- Was your interpretation correct?
- What confirmed that it was correct?
- If it was not correct, what evidence did you have that it was not correct?
- What did you base your subsequent decision on?
- How did you know it was the right decision?

As this activity is based on your personal experiences, there is an outline answer to only part of this activity at the end of the chapter.

Being confident enough to communicate the evidence base for your actions to others is often subject to the atmospheres that can exist in the workplace or the classroom. Lack of managerial or tutor support in situations can reduce cooperation and can promote organisational friction. It is important to analyse critically surrounding factors such as leadership and your responses to it in order to identify facilitative and hindering factors that may also affect situations and decision making.

Scenario: A case of dealing with pressure

Arunda was a student in the second year of her nurse preparation programme. She was working in an **endoscopy** *suite. The unit was short staffed and had many complex patients to deal with. Although Arunda was supposed to be supernumerary, she had to work as a regular member of staff to help them deal with the complex patients. One in particular caused her concern. The patient was an alcoholic and attended*

---

continued . . .

for an **oesophagealgastroduedonoscopy (OGD)** *procedure. The results showed that he had oesophageal varices, which are enlarged veins at the base of the oesophagus. Arunda was responsible for monitoring his vital signs. The patient started to bleed. Arunda alerted the team that the vital signs were changing. Stabilising the patient took some time. Afterwards Arunda helped to clean and decontaminate the equipment. Arunda and the team went off duty late. Just before they were leaving the manager praised Arunda, telling her she had done a good job. The following week Arunda asked her mentor if she could take back some of the time she had used staying behind to help with the emergency. She wanted to see her daughter's school play. The manager was on holiday at the time and Arunda's mentor (who had not been present at the emergency) refused, saying Arunda still had a lot to learn in her last week. Arunda met with her university link tutor who asked her how her placement had been. Arunda said it had been tough but she had learned a lot.*

Questions
- What sources of evidence might Arunda use to evaluate her learning?
- What sources of evidence was the manager using to evaluate Arunda's learning?
- What sources of evidence was the mentor using to evaluate Arunda's learning?

There are outline answers to these questions at the end of the chapter.

When interpretations are not checked for their validity it is possible for our fears and anxieties to become projected on to another person or situation, and for us to interact with that person or situation as if they meant us harm. Critical reflection helps to make sense of the evidence supporting the validity of our interpretations and how ideas fit together. We proceed now to consider how new ideas come together within critical reflection.

Identifying the coming together of new ideas

Critical reflection offers you psychological space to connect with your ideas and those of others, as well as the mental focus to do so. Your ideas and knowledge may be diverse, but you need also to be open to challenge in order to progress. In essence, this means drawing together ideas of process, building relationships, caring and ethical behaviours to inform the practice of nursing. Nursing knowledge, in this sense, is something interconnected and emerging as a discipline in its own right while you, as a practitioner, work out your ideas and contribute to knowledge within practice. This role of authorship continues reflexive dialogue with the ideas obtained from external sources as you progress through your nurse preparation course if you are a novice practitioner, or through your nursing career if you are an experienced practitioner. In this way you develop agency as you also focus on possible further development needs.

However, lack of feedback also reduces the possibility of developing ideas. Therefore, discussing your critical reflections is a really important component of bringing new ideas together. While you are on your nurse preparation course you will need the support of mentors, tutors and clinical colleagues to be able to develop new ideas of how to act in the future. Even if you are an experienced practitioner, you will still need the support of colleagues to challenge and discuss your practice in positive ways. Ideas can become 'worked out' and criticality and imagination awakened. Becoming proactive in looking for ideas, rather than simply accepting them, is an important step towards building imagination and learning that is more long-lasting and critical.

How ideas from the different ways of reflecting that have been discussed throughout this book are brought together, or not, is illustrated in Figure 11.1.

The outer world encompasses learning that is generated by political systems, organisational structures and scientific enquiry, and that is represented by codified knowledge. This learning can be associated with the guidance that delivers it, to be internally considered. For example, your mentors and teachers will identify what you need to learn, give you information and direct you to complete learning tasks. If you are an experienced practitioner you may be engaging with continuing professional development (CPD) courses. But it is only you who can make real sense of what this means to you and what you are taking forward through what I term 'inner world consideration'.

Political, cognitive, scientific and professional ideas are all consistent with outer world experiences that intrude on the personal world, where they are met by inner world sense making. The interface between your outer and inner world experience is porous in that it allows experiences and learning to interact. The inner world encompasses critical learning that helps to internalise experiences, and that may also be influential in shaping new ones, for example in the level of self-confidence a person has or the quality of their self-esteem. This inner world includes biographical, personal and emotional dimensions and reflexive, imaginative and creative responses

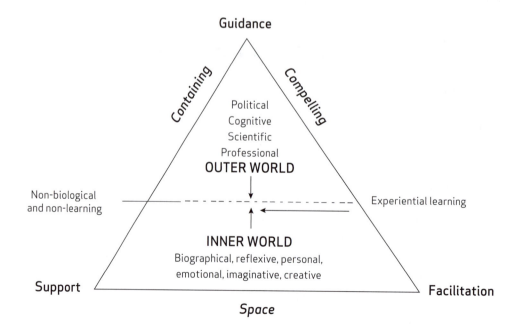

Figure 11.1: Inter-relationships between inner and outer worlds of learning and containing and compelling space
Source: Howatson-Jones (2010).

to these dimensions. It is also where your values are embedded. These might relate to the continuous internal dialogue that you have with yourself in response to what is happening externally; your emotional life, which influences your reactions; and maybe biographical memories, which are a part of your sense making.

Experiential learning is located at the interface between inner and outer worlds, as it is here that outer and inner world experiences become worked through in either direction. In other words, your internal world can influence the outer world experiences you find yourself in and vice versa. For example, consider that you are a spontaneous creative person (inner world). Finding yourself in situations where others are constantly organising you and telling you what you must do and learn can feel constricting and oppressive (outer world). You want to learn to be a professional nurse so some compromise needs to be reached at the experiential interface between these two worlds. This is where facilitation and support are crucial.

The biographical, personal and emotional dimensions, and reflexive, imaginative and creative responses to these dimensions are influenced by the qualities of facilitation and support and how these qualities may be included or excluded from learning opportunities in spaces that are more or less containing and compelling. Such a space links guidance, facilitation and support to help contain anxiety and make learning manageable. Where these are lacking, the interface between inner and outer worlds becomes less porous and more rigid, with little chance of critical reflection taking place. The result is non-biographical learning, where nothing is perceived as new but instead information is just processed with non-awareness and a lack of openness, so that experiences may be gathered, but nothing learned from them. Consider the following case study to make sense of these processes.

Case study: Cassie's difficulty with saying no

Cassie was a newly qualified nurse working on a gynaecology ward, which she loved. She had previously been a care worker in a care home before undertaking her nursing preparation programme. Cassie had always been hard-working and had completed tasks to a very high standard. Consequently, the nursing home manager had come to rely on Cassie and had frequently asked her to help out when others would not. Cassie had felt flattered to be needed and had complied, even though the extra workload often made her feel stressed and put a strain on family life.

Cassie had undertaken her nurse preparation programme with the blessing of her family. Throughout the programme, she had tried to maintain her family role and study hard. At one stage she did think of quitting because of the strain everything was putting on her. Fortunately, she contacted her tutor, who met with her and encouraged Cassie to reflect on what she was doing. This helped Cassie to realise that she was taking a passive role, rather than exerting some agency in her life. She did not want to be thought of badly by her family or by her colleagues.

In her present role as a newly registered nurse, Cassie decided that she needed some help to overcome the hurdles she was experiencing of having to solve many problem issues that were unfamiliar. Cassie decided to access clinical supervision, which was offered by her employer. At the first session her clinical supervisor,

continued . . .

Annie, asked Cassie to reflect on her journey from being a care worker to becoming a qualified nurse. Together Cassie and Annie critically examined Cassie's approach to work and noted her tendency to overwork and not be able to say no. Following through the consequences highlighted to Cassie how she was not learning from what she was experiencing, but instead was trying to conform to others' views. Through Annie's positive guidance Cassie felt confident enough to acknowledge to herself that she was not a bad person, or nurse, if at times she said no. In fact, this might sometimes be the responsible thing to do. Cassie continued to reflect long after leaving the session and was more considered in approaching problems and caring for herself as a result.

While reflection may be able to vent some of the emotional residues of your work, the critical element is vital in order to avoid becoming snared in narcissistic contemplation that does not move you, or your learning, forward. Interrogating the line between inner and outer world experience is where awareness of new ideas springs from, and is where you can become aware of what you are learning and how to exert some agency within it.

Chapter summary

Critical reflection is part of being a responsible and accountable practitioner, by examining and analysing your practice and learning. As has been noted in this chapter, it requires discipline and systematic thought in order to interrogate what you are doing and the evidence base of your interpretations and decisions. These aspects can be missed from simple reflection on practice, which concentrates on feeling elements. Through the activities in this chapter, you have been offered an opportunity to complete the cycle of connecting feelings, evidence, decisions and actions through critical reflection that takes an analytical view of your practice and development.

Activities and scenarios: Brief outline answers

Activity 11.1: Critical thinking (page 147)

The incident or event you might have described could have been a mistake or an accident, or something that went particularly well, such as therapeutic communication. You are likely to have identified the importance of the event in developing your practice. Feelings will have depended on whether you viewed the event as positive or negative. For example, a mistake is likely to have created feelings of acute anxiety, while receiving a compliment from a patient is likely to have elicited feelings of confidence. Satisfactory elements are likely to have been related to your actions that were affirmed by others and to positive responses from patients. Concerning elements would have arisen where you were uncertain of what to do and of others' responses to you, for example if you were shouted at or told you were wrong. What you could do differently would probably relate to improving your knowledge, finding out the facts of the case, seeking help and considering how you use communication. Additional knowledge you might have needed could relate to policies and procedures. The learning that you might take forward is potentially going to relate to communication and decision making, as well as knowing more about yourself and how you respond to situations.

Activity 11.3: Critical thinking (page 152)

The sources of evidence that you might have used are likely to have included the following.

- Objective and subjective data to base your assessment on, such as what you found out through communication, what you observed, what you felt, practice policies and theoretical ideas.
- Communication and observation are likely to have confirmed whether your interpretation was correct or identified deficits.
- You might have based your decision making on a protocol, or an assessment of the alternatives and possible consequences, or on intuition or what you had read.
- How you knew it was the right decision would have been through the feedback of others and what you observed the consequences to be.

Scenario: Integrating a new member of staff (page 149)

As the experienced member of staff perhaps I should have negotiated expectations more plainly at the start, and identified sources of information more clearly. Perhaps I need to give more feedback to help boost her confidence. Maybe I am more controlling than I think. I am used to working autonomously and therefore difficulties seem to have arisen from a need for adjustment. I realise I have very high personal standards and am very competent, and therefore have similar expectations from others, which might be threatening. I feel my management style is democratic, but my standards and expectations may be a controlling influence. Giving more feedback may help to negate her anxious behaviours. Identifying sources of information and outlining organisational and personal needs may help to clarify concerns.

As a new member of staff, I do feel very anxious about getting things right. I have tried to arrange to work hours that are mutually manageable. I am trying to develop my skills through experiencing as much as I can with the support of others, making sure I am doing things right. But I feel they think I am a nuisance. I can see that the clinical area is very busy. I need to consider the needs of colleagues as well as my own in order to be effective. Discussing expectations and feedback arrangements might help both parties to find mutually acceptable solutions to my childcare commitments as well as work requirements.

Scenario: Fajid's understanding of young carers (page 151)

Fajid assumes that health and social care are the same thing. He does not understand that there are costs attached to social care. These are financial as well as personal. Social care needs to be paid for. Some people are also reluctant to have strangers caring for them, especially when it involves personal care. It is natural for Kate to want to help her mother. However, taking on too much is likely to impact on her socially and educationally. Equally, if Fajid is not knowledgeable about why children become carers and about available resources he cannot help Kate's mother to make different choices as she is the adult in this situation.

Scenario: A case of dealing with pressure (pages 152–3)

Arunda might use the evidence of recognising the significance of vital sign changes to demonstrate her knowledge of physiology. She could also consider the manager's praise of a job well done as showing she can work well under pressure. The manager was using Arunda's ability to stay calm under pressure and report changes accurately as evidence that Arunda had embedded knowledge. However, this is only in a narrow field and would not necessarily evaluate all the learning that was required of her in this placement. The mentor is likely to be taking a broader view and may be using the criteria in the assessment of practice learning to evaluate Arunda's learning. She may consider Arunda's request to go home early as evidence that she does not want to learn.

Further reading

Cottrell, S (2011) *Critical Thinking Skills: Developing effective analysis and argument*, 2nd edition. Basingstoke: Palgrave.

This book can help you to develop the analysis techniques that are a necessary part of critical reflection.

Metcalfe, M (2006) *Reading Critically at University.* Los Angeles, CA: Sage.

This book can help you to develop understanding of how to review critically sources of information and learning.

Whitehead, DK, Weiss, SA and Tappen, RM (2007) *Essentials of Nursing Leadership and Management*, 4th edition. Philadelphia, PA: FA Davis.

This book can help you to use critical thought in developing in your role, and in developing leadership and management skills.

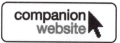

For further activities and other useful material, visit the companion website at **www.sagepub.co.uk/howatson-jones_reflective2e**

Glossary

agency: how a person makes use of their life resources to develop strategies for change.

analgesia: medication that eases pain.

aortic stent insertion: a plastic tube that is inserted into the aorta to keep the vessel patent and protect the wall of the vessel.

becoming: a process of change that alters a sense of personal identity.

benign MS: a mild form of multiple sclerosis (MS) experienced by approx 10 per cent of sufferers.

catalytic: prompting deep exploration and analysis.

cathartic: prompting the release of emotion.

clonic: descriptive of the jerky movements resulting from muscular spasms.

compelling space: a space that invites a desire to learn in more meaningful ways.

culture: the meanings and understandings held by a group of people that influence the way they think and act.

cyanosed: having a lack of oxygen in the tissues, evidenced by a bluish tinge to the lips and fingernails.

ectopic pregnancy: a fertilised egg that has lodged in the fallopian tube and that is at risk of rupturing the tube as it grows.

empowerment: taking personal control.

endoscopy: a procedure that visualises the inside of body cavities and tracts using camera technology with a light source and a steerable flexible tube.

epileptic fit: a seizure that can manifest itself in a variety of ways and that is caused by electrical disruption in the brain.

haemorrhoidectomy: removal of haemorrhoids, which are swollen blood vessels usually located in the anal area.

health promotion: encouraging people to examine and change their lifestyles to ones that are healthy.

intuition / intuitive knowledge: experience-based knowledge.

learning contract: a plan of learning objectives agreed between the student and their supervisor.

learning style: a preference for particular ways of learning.

lifeworld: the history, culture, situations and relationships of an individual.

losing face: feeling a loss of respect.

metastases: spread of cells and disease (usually cancer) to another part of the body.

multiple sclerosis (MS): incurable neurological condition caused by destruction of the insulation layer surrounding some nerves, which results in disruption of the nerve pathways.

oesophagealgastroduodenoscopy (OGD): a procedure where a flexible tube with a camera is passed through the oesophagus, stomach and duodenum to visualise the internal lining and structure.

oncology: cancer care.

phlebitis: inflammation of a vein.

reflection: considering and reviewing thinking, actions and circumstances to develop new ideas.

reflective cycle: a cyclical structuring of consideration and review of thinking, actions and circumstances to develop new ideas.

reflective framework: framing structuring of consideration and review of thinking, actions and circumstances with questions.

reflective practice: considering and reviewing the interplay between theory and practice and new ideas.

reflexivity: the conscious engagement on the part of the practitioner to being open to examining their own assumptions and influences on situations, and how the cultures and contexts they are embedded in might be influencing them.

self-concept: a perception of who one is and of personal capability.

socialisation: socialisation is a process of developing meaning through interaction and adaptation.

Skype: Skype allows the user to communicate over the internet using voice or video contact so that you can see each other face to face.

tacit knowledge: knowledge that is so deeply embedded that people often forget they have it. It is known to people within a group and does not need explanation within the context of that group, but may be unknown to outsiders.

tonic: descriptive of muscle rigidity.

transitional space: where a person is able to consider and try out other ways of being.

Trust: management unit of NHS healthcare, which may encompass a number of providers and settings.

uterine embolisation: deliberate occlusion of the uterine arteries to terminate blood flow.

venepuncture: taking a blood sample from a vein.

wiki: electronic tool for organising information.

References

Abrahamson, CE (1998) Storytelling as a pedagogical tool in higher education. *Education*, 118(3): 440–51.

Abrandt Dahlgren, M, Richardson, B and Kalman, H (2004) Redefining the reflective practitioner, in Higgs, J, Richardson, B and Abrandt Dahlgren, M (eds) *Developing Practice Knowledge for Health Professionals.* Edinburgh: Butterworth Heinemann, pp15–34.

Alheit, P and Dausien, B (2007) Lifelong learning and biography: a competitive dynamic between the macro- and the micro-level of education, in West, L, Alheit, P, Andersen Siig, A and Merrill, B (eds) *Using Biographical and Life History Approaches in the Study of Adult and Lifelong Learning: European perspectives.* Frankfurt am Main: Peter Lang, pp57–70.

Andrew, N, Tolson, D and Ferguson, D (2008) Building on Wenger: communities of practice in nursing. *Nurse Education Today*, 28: 246–52.

Argyris, C and Schön, D (1978) *Organisational Learning: A theory of action perspective.* Reading, MA: Addison-Wesley.

Armitage, G (2009) The risks of double checking. *Nursing Management*, 16(2): 30–5.

Atkins, S and Murphy, K (1995) Reflective practice. *Nursing Standard*, 9(45): 31–7.

Benner, P (1984) *From Novice to Expert: Excellence and power in clinical nursing practice.* Menlo Park, CA: Addison-Wesley.

Bishop, V (2007) *Clinical Supervision in Practice*, 2nd edition. Basingstoke: Palgrave Macmillan.

Boase, C (2008) *Digital Storytelling for Reflection and Engagement: A study of the uses and potential of digital storytelling.* Available online at http://resources.glos.ac.uk/shareddata/dms/766118A3BCD42A03921A19B460003 A91.doc (accessed 8 August 2012).

Bohinc, M and Gradisar, M (2003) Decision-making model for nursing. *Journal of Nursing Administration*, 33(12): 627–9.

Bolton, G (2010) *Reflective Practice: Writing and professional development*, 3rd edition. Los Angeles, CA: Sage.

Boud, D and Miller, N (1996) *Working with Experience: Animating learning.* London: Routledge.

Boud, D, Keogh, R and Walker, D (eds) (1985) *Reflection: Turning experience into learning.* London: Kogan Page.

Brechin, A (2000) Introducing critical practice, in Brechin, A, Brown, H and Eby, A (eds) *Critical Practice in Health and Social Care.* London: Sage, pp25–47.

Brockbank, A and McGill, I (1998) *Facilitating Reflective Learning in Higher Education.* Buckingham: Society for Research into Higher Education/Open University Press.

Brookfield, S (2005) *The Power of Critical Theory for Adult Learning and Teaching.* Maidenhead: Open University Press.

Bulman, C and Schutz, S (eds) (2008) *Reflective Practice in Nursing*, 4th edition. Oxford: Blackwell Science.

Carper, B (1978) Fundamental patterns of knowing in nursing. *Advances in Nursing Science*, 1(1): 13–23.

Cassidy, S (2009) Interpretation of competence in student assessment. *Nursing Standard*, 23(18): 39–46.

Chan, EA and Schwind, JK (2006) Two teachers reflect on acquiring their nursing identity. *Reflective Practice*, 7(3): 303–14.

Chirema, KD (2007) The use of reflective journals in the promotion of reflection and learning in post-registration nursing students. *Nurse Education Today*, 27: 192–202.

Crabtree, BF (2003) Primary care practices are full of surprises. *Health Care Management Review*, 28(3): 275–83.

Curzon-Hobson, A (2002) A pedagogy of trust in higher learning. *Teaching in Higher Education*, 7(3): 265–76.

Daley, B (2001) Learning in clinical nursing practice. *Holistic Nursing Practice*, 16(1): 43–54.

Dalton, D (2005) Dyslexics should not be discriminated against. *Nursing Standard*, 19(36): 39.

Davis, N, Clark, AC, O'Brien, M, Plaice, C, Sumpton, K and Waugh, S (2011) *Learning Skills for Nursing Students*. Exeter: Learning Matters.

Department of Health (DH) (1997) *The Caldicott Committee Report on the Review of Patient Identifiable Information*. London: HMSO.

Department of Health (DH) (2008a) *High Quality Care for All*. London: HMSO.

Department of Health (DH) (2008b) *A High Quality Workforce*. London: HMSO.

Department of Health (DH) (2009) *The NHS Constitution: Securing the NHS today for generations to come*. London: HMSO.

Dix, G and Hughes, SJ (2004) Strategies to help students learn effectively. *Nursing Standard*, 18(32): 39–42.

Dominice, P (2000) *Learning from Ourselves*. San Francisco, CA: Jossey-Bass.

Driscoll, J (2007) *Practising Clinical Supervision: A reflective approach for healthcare professionals*, second revised edition. Edinburgh: Bailliere Tindall.

Ehrmann, G (2005) Managing the aggressive nursing student. *Nurse Educator*, 30(3): 98–100.

Ellis, P (2013) *Evidence-based Practice in Nursing*, 2nd edition. London: Sage.

Ellis, P and Howatson-Jones, L (2008) Conclusion, in Howatson-Jones, L and Ellis, P (eds) (2008) *Outpatient, Day Surgery and Ambulatory Care*. Chichester: Wiley-Blackwell.

Eraut, M (2001) *Developing Professional Knowledge and Competence*, 2nd edition. London: The Falmer Press.

Falconer, L (2011) Upload and update. *Nursing Standard*, 25(31): 26–7.

Faugier, J and Butterworth, T (1994) *Clinical Supervision: A position paper*. Manchester: University of Manchester.

Field, J (2006) *Lifelong Learning and the New Educational Order*, 2nd edition. Stoke-on-Trent: Trentham Books.

Fischer-Rosenthal, W (2000) Biographical work and biographical structuring in present-day stories, in Chamberlayne, P, Bornat, J and Wengraf, T (eds) *The Turn to Biographical Methods in Social Science: Comparative issues and examples*. London and New York: Routledge, pp109–25.

Freshwater, D (2000) Crosscurrents: against cultural narration in nursing. *Journal of Advanced Nursing*, 32(2): 481–4.

Ghaye, T and Lillyman, S (2010) *Reflection: Principles and practice for healthcare professionals*, 2nd edition. Dinton: Quay Books/Mark Allen.

Gibbs, G (1988) *Learning By Doing: A guide to teaching and learning methods*, RP 391. London: FEU.

Glaze, JE (2001) Stages in coming to terms with reflection: student advanced nurse practitioners' perceptions of their reflective journeys. *Journal of Advanced Nursing* 37 (3): 263–72.

Hargreaves, J (1997) Using patients: exploring the ethical dimension of reflective practice in nurse education. *Journal of Advanced Nursing*, 25(2): 223–8.

Hinchliff, S, Norman, S and Schober, J (2008) *Nursing Practice and Health Care: A foundation text*, 5th edition. London: Hodder Arnold.

Holmes, J (2005) Notes on mentalizing – old hat, or new wine? *British Journal of Psychotherapy*, 22(2): 179–97.

Horowitz, SA (2004) The discovery and loss of a 'compelling space': a case study in adapting to a new organisational order, in Huffington, C, Armstrong, D, Halton, W, Hoyle, L and Pooley, J (eds) *Working Below the Surface: The emotional life of contemporary organisations*. London: Karnac, pp151–63.

Horsdal, M (2007) Therapy and narratives of self, in West, L, Alheit, P, Anderson, AS and Merill, B (eds) *Using Biographical and Life History Approaches in the Study of Adult and Lifelong Learning: European perspectives*. Frankfurt am Main: Peter Lang, pp187–203.

Horsdal, M (2012) *Telling Lives: Exploring dimensions of narratives*. London: Routledge.

Howatson-Jones, L (2003) Difficulties in clinical supervision and lifelong learning. *Nursing Standard*, 17(37): 37–41.

Howatson-Jones, L (2010) *Exploring the Learning of Nurses*, unpublished PhD thesis. Canterbury: Canterbury Christ Church University/University of Kent.

Hunt, C and West, L (2007) Salvaging the self in adult learning: auto/biographical perspectives from teaching and research. Paper presented at the Conference of the ESREA Network on Life History and Biography. Denmark: Roskilde University.

Hutchfield, K (2010) *Information Skills for Nursing Students*. Exeter: Learning Matters.

Iedema, R (2011) Creating safety by strengthening clinicians' capacity for reflexivity. *British Medical Journal Quality & Safety*, 20(suppl. 1): i83–i86. Doi: 10.1136/bmjqs.2010.046714.

Illeris, K (2004) *The Three Dimensions of Learning: Contemporary learning theory in the tension field between cognitive, the emotional and the social*, 2nd edition. Roskilde: Roskilde University Press and NIACE.

Jacques, D (2000) *Learning in Groups*, 3rd edition. London: Kogan Page.

Jarvis, P (2006) *Towards a Comprehensive Theory of Human Learning*, Lifelong Learning and the Learning Society, volume 1. London: Routledge.

Jarvis, P (2007) *Globalisation, Lifelong Learning and the Learning Society: Sociological perspectives*, Lifelong Learning and the Learning Society, volume 2. Abingdon: Routledge.

Jarvis, P (2010) *Adult Education and Lifelong Learning: Theory and practice*, 4th edition. New York: Routledge.

Jasper, M (2003) *Beginning Reflective Practice*. Cheltenham: Nelson Thornes.

Johns, C (1995) Framing learning through reflection within Carper's fundamental ways of knowing in nursing. *Journal of Advanced Nursing*, 22: 226–34.

Johns, C (1997) Reflective practice and clinical supervision – part 1: the reflective turn. *European Nurse*, 2(2): 87–97.

Johns, C (2002) *Guided Reflection: Advancing practice*. Oxford: Blackwell Science.

Johns, C (2004) *Becoming a Reflective Practitioner*, 2nd edition. Oxford: Blackwell.

Johns, C (2007) Deep in reflection. *Nursing Standard*, 21(38): 24–5.

Johns, C (2009) *Becoming a Reflective Practitioner*, 3rd edition. Chichester: Blackwell.

Johns, C (2010) *Guided Reflection: A narrative approach to advancing professional practice*, 2nd edition. Chichester: Wiley-Blackwell.

Johns, C and Freshwater, D (eds) (2005) *Transforming Nursing through Reflective Practice*, 2nd edition. Oxford: Blackwell.

Kozlowski, D (2002) Using online learning in a traditional face-to-face environment. *Computers in Nursing*, 20(1): 23–30.

Lee, NJ (2009) Using group reflection in an action research study. *Nurse Researcher*, 16(1): 30–42.

Lindsay, GM (2006) Constructing a nursing identity: reflecting on and reconstructing experience. *Reflective Practice*, 7(1): 59–72.

Lynch, L, Hancox, K, Happell, B and Parker, J (2008) *Clinical Supervision for Nurses*. Chichester: Wiley-Blackwell.

Maich, NM, Brown, B and Royle, J (2000) 'Becoming' through reflection and professional portfolios: the voice of growth in nurses. *Reflective Practice*, 1(6). Available online at http://ejournals.ebsco.com (accessed 23 July 2007).

Mason-Whitehead, E and Mason, T (2008) *Study Skills for Nurses*, 2nd edition. Los Angeles, CA: Sage.

Matthews-DeNatale, G (2008) *Digital Story Telling: Tips and resources*. Available online at http://net.educause.edu/ir/library/pdf/ELI08167B.pdf (accessed 8 August 2012).

Milne, D (2009) *Evidence-based Clinical Supervision: Principles and practice*. Oxford: British Psychological Society and Blackwell.

Morton-Cooper, A and Palmer, A (2000) *Mentoring, Preceptorship and Clinical Supervision: A guide to professional support roles in clinical practice*, 2nd edition. Oxford: Blackwell.

Muir, N (2004) Clinical decision-making: theory and practice. *Nursing Standard*, 18(36): 47–52.

Nursing and Midwifery Council (NMC) (2006) *Clinical Supervision*. London: NMC. Available online at www.nmc-uk.org/aFrameDisplay.aspx?DocumentID=1558 (accessed 28 September 2007).

Nursing and Midwifery Council (NMC) (2008) *The Code: Standards of conduct, performance and ethics for nurses and midwives*. London: NMC.

Nursing and Midwifery Council (2010a) *Standards for Pre-registration Nursing Education*. London: NMC.

Nursing and Midwifery Council (2010b) *Guidance on Professional Conduct for Nursing and Midwifery Students*, 2nd edition. London: NMC.

Nursing and Midwifery Council (2012) *Social Networking Sites*. Available online at www.nmc-uk.org/Nurses-and-midwives/Advice-by-topic/A/Advice/Social-networking-sites (accessed 26 July 2012).

Ohler, J (2008) *Digital Storytelling in the Classroom: New media pathways to literacy, learning and creativity*. Thousand Oaks, CA: Corwin Press.

Ousey, K and Johnson, M (2007) Being a real nurse: concepts of caring and culture in the clinical areas. *Nurse Education in Practice*, 7(3): 150–5.

Palmer, A, Burns, S and Bulman, C (1994) *Reflective Practice in Nursing: The growth of the Professional Practitioner*. Oxford: Blackwell Scientific.

Parse, RR (1998) *The Human Becoming School of Thought*, 2nd edition. Thousand Oaks, CA: Sage.

Percival, J (2001) Know your enemy. *Nursing Standard*, 15(35): 24–5.

Petty, G (2009) *Teaching Today: A practical guide*, 4th edition. Cheltenham: Nelson Thornes.

Phelan, A, Barlow, C and Iversen, S (2006) Occasioning learning in the workplace: the case of interprofessional peer collaboration. *Journal of Interprofessional Care*, 20(4): 415–24.

Pierson, W (1998) Reflection and nursing education. *Journal of Advanced Nursing*, 27: 165–70.

Price, B (2008) The intelligent workforce. *Nursing Management*, 15(5): 28–33.

Proctor, B (1986) Supervision: a co-operative exercise in accountability, in Hawkins, P and Shohet, R (eds) (1989) *Supervision in the Helping Professions*. Milton Keynes: Open University Press.

Quality Assurance Agency (QAA) (2008) *The Framework for Higher Education Qualifications in England, Wales and Northern Ireland*. Mansfield: QAA.

Reed, S (2011) *Successful Professional Portfolios for Nursing Students*. Exeter: Learning Matters.

Richardson, L (1997) *Fields of Play: Constructing an academic life*. New Brunswick, NJ: Rutgers University Press.

Rogers, C and Freiberg, HJ (1994) *Freedom to Learn*, 3rd edition. New York: Macmillan College.

Rolfe, G (ed.) (2011) *Critical Reflection in Practice: Generating knowledge for caring*, 2nd edition. Basingstoke: Palgrave.

Royal College of Nursing (RCN) (2009) *Legal Advice for RCN Members Using the Internet*. London: RCN. Available online at www.rcn.org.uk/__data/assets/pdf_file/0008/272195/003557.pdf (accessed 8 August 2012).

Royal College of Nursing (RCN) (2011) *Social Networking and Nursing*. Available online at www.rcn.org.uk/ newsevents/congress/congress_2011/congress_2011_agenda/9._social_networking_and_nursing (accessed 26 July 2012).

Scanlan, J and Chernomas, W (1997) Developing the reflective teacher. *Journal of Advanced Nursing*, 25(6): 1138–43.

Schmidt, NA (2008) Guided imagery as internally orientated self-care: a nursing case. *Self-care, Dependent-care and Nursing*, 16(1): 41–8. Available online at http://web.ebscohost.com/ehost/pdf?vid=30&hid= 108&sid=976025b3-798d-4793-a2ee-c056432c1363%40sessionmgr104 (accessed 19 September 2009).

Schön, D (1987) *Educating the Reflective Practitioner: Toward a new design for teaching and learning in the professions*. San Francisco, CA: Jossey-Bass.

Schön, D (1991) *The Reflective Practitioner: How professionals think in action*. Farnham: Arena, Ashgate.

Sennett, R (2008) *The Craftsman*. London: Allen Lane/Penguin Books.

Smith, A and Jack, K (2005) Reflective practice: a meaningful task for students. *Nursing Standard*, 19(26): 33–7.

Spinks, M (2009) Compassion in care. *Nursing Management*, 16(5): 11.

Sully, P and Dallas, J (2005) *Essential Communication Skills for Nursing*. Edinburgh: Elsevier Mosby.

Tappen, RM, Weiss, SA and Whitehead, DK (2004) *Essentials of Nursing Leadership and Management*, 3rd edition. Philadelphia, PA: FA Davis.

Taylor, B (2010) *Reflective Practice for Healthcare Professionals*, 3rd edition. Maidenhead: Open University Press.

Thompson, C and Dowding, D (eds) (2002) *Clinical Decision-making and Judgement in Nursing*. Edinburgh: Churchill Livingstone.

Thorndycraft, B and McCabe, J (2008) The challenge of working with staff groups in the caring professions: the importance of the 'Team Development and Reflective Practice Group'. *British Journal of Psychotherapy*, 24(2): 167–82.

Titchen, A and McGinley, M, with McCormack, B (2004) Blending self-knowledge and professional knowledge, in Higgs, J, Richardson, B and Abrandt Dahlgren, M (eds) *Developing Practice Knowledge for Health Professionals*. Edinburgh: Butterworth Heinemann, pp107–26.

Twigg, J (2006) *The Body in Health and Social Care.* Basingstoke: Palgrave Macmillan.

United Kingdom Central Council (UKCC) for Nursing, Midwifery and Health Visiting (1994) *The Future of Professional Practice: The Council's standard for education and practice following registration.* London: UKCC.

van Boven, L, White, K, Kamada, A and Gilovich, T (2003) Intuitions about situational correction in self and others. *Journal of Personality and Social Psychology,* 85(2): 249–58.

van Ooijen, E (2003) *Clinical Supervision Made Easy.* Edinburgh: Churchill Livingstone.

Watson, J (1985) *Nursing: The philosophy and science of caring.* Boulder, CO: Associated University Press.

Watson, J (1988) *Nursing: Human Science and Human Care: A theory of nursing.* New York: National League for Nursing.

Wenger, E (1998) *Communities of Practice: Learning, meaning and identity.* Cambridge: Cambridge University Press.

West, L (2001) *Doctors on the Edge: General practitioners' health and learning in the inner city.* London: Free Associates Books.

West, L, Alheit, P, Anderson, AS and Merill, B (2007) (eds) *Using Biographical and Life History Approaches in the Study of Adult and Lifelong Learning: European perspectives.* Frankfurt am Main: Peter Lang.

Winnicott, DW (1965) *The Maturational Processes and the Facilitating Environment: Studies in the theory of emotional development.* London: Karnac and the Institute of Psycho-Analysis.

Xu, Y and Davidhizar, R (2005) Intercultural communication in nursing education: when Asian students and American faculty converge. *Journal of Nursing Education,* 44(5): 209–15.

Zander, PE (2007) Ways of knowing in nursing: the historical evolution of a concept. *Journal of Theory Construction and Testing,* 11(1): 7–11. Available online at http://web.ebscohost.com/ehost/pdf?vid=6&hid=105&sid=3c39801a-fa7b-47e2-b6cb-c946e9680d65%40sessionmgr113 (accessed 20 December 2009).

Index